2 W[EEKS]

in the

F∧ST

LANE

DIET

Fiona Kirk

for more information visit
www.fionakirk.com

Painless Publishing

Published in the UK 2011 by **Painless Publishing**

www.painlesspublishing.com

Note to Readers

If you are pregnant, breastfeeding, on regular medication, have concerns about your health or are under the age of 16 you should consult your doctor or health practitioner before embarking on any new eating and/or exercise programme. Every effort has been made to present the information in this book in a clear, complete and accurate manner, however not every situation can be anticipated and the information in this book cannot take the place of a medical analysis of individual health needs. The author and Painless Publishing hereby disclaim any and all liability resulting from injuries or damage caused by following any recommendations in this book.

References

All statements (other than personal views) and studies referred to throughout the book have been exhaustively researched but the author chose not to reference them throughout the text and add copious additional pages at the back of the book. Should you wish further information about any of the above, email through the author's website www.fionakirk.com and they will be provided promptly.

Recipes

All recipes serve 1 or 2 people. Adapt according to required portion numbers.

Typesetting/Cover Design **Katy Buchan**
Images **Isla Munro**
Chapter Introductions **Liam Smith**

148pp
ISBN 978 0 9566115 1 2

About Me

I get very passionate about stuff and can rant for hours if given the chance! Dieting and fat loss are often at the top of my hit list. Why? Because I believe that anyone can lose weight and keep it off without having to stick to a rigid regime that takes all the fun out of eating and find a route that suits. Our lifestyles, our preferences, our tastes and our crazy indulgences make each and every one of us totally individual and when we recognise, understand and embrace them we can create a way of eating that works and permanent fat loss follows.

Am I slim? Yes. Am I fit? Reasonably. Do I follow a diet? Yes and no. Yes, because I have, after a lot of research, hit upon a way of eating that keeps my body nourished, gives me the energy to fulfil my often onerous daily commitments and allows me to sleep like a baby most nights. No, because **I refuse to deprive myself of the things I love**. I love to

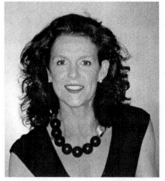

cook, I love to experiment with new and exciting ways to prepare and present delicious dishes, I love to party (and food is generally involved!) but perhaps most importantly, **I love food in all its guises** and refuse to let the food police dictate what I should be eating and when. They don't live my life, I do!

Have I always been slim? No. Have I always been fit? When I was young, yes. Have I experimented with loads of diets? Yes. Did any of them work? Short term, mostly yes, long term, no. So what changed? I went back to school at the ripe old age of forty-something, learned a lot about nutrition and health and after four long years of study, followed by another four or five long years of trial and error worked out what works for me. I rediscovered my waistline, climbed into a pair of ridiculously skinny jeans and have never looked back. My mission in this canny little diet book is to present you with a 14 day programme that can achieve fast fat loss and continued fat loss. Ignore what you may have read or heard about diets failing to achieve long term and read on!

NB: I don't intend to add copious pages to this book by explaining the biochemical intricacies of blood sugar balance, the importance of macro and micro nutrients for energy, repair and regeneration or why many diets are doomed to failure from the start. This is simply a handbag/briefcase-sized book about the way forward. Fat loss forever. However, I am a big fan of anyone who wants to know more and if you are that kind of animal, go onto my website and nab yourself a copy of my book *So What the F*** Should I Eat?* which explains all. www.fionakirk.com

And Another Thing...
Whilst I have endeavoured to make this book an easy read, it is impossible to pass on some of the important messages without resorting to the use of technical nutritional terms on occasion. There is a glossary at the back of the book - refer to it whenever you come across any words/principles that require further explanation and if you want more information, email me through my website. The aim is to cut through the confusion not add to it!

What they said about...
*So What the F*** Should I Eat?*

"What I most like about Fiona is her ability to distil complicated nutritional advice into no-nonsense, down to earth language that everyone can understand. Even better, her warmth, wit and wisdom come shining through on every page. If you want to lose weight and more importantly keep it off, Fiona is the nutritionist for you."
Dan Roberts, the Wellbeing Coach www.danroberts.com

"We reviewed Fiona's book, So what the F*** Should I Eat? on site back in November 2010 and concluded 'This isn't just some sort of cheer leading exercise promising the moon on a stick, rather a realistic way to change your health and well-being for the better.' Since then Fiona has become a valued member of the Foodepedia team, supplying us with reviews of some of the restaurants she has visited in Scotland. Fiona's approach to diet rather than 'dieting' is refreshing and encouraging to us all. Enjoying good food while making careful choices about those foods that we all know are heavily calorific is absolutely the way to go."
Alan King, Deputy Editor, www.foodepedia.co.uk

"I love Fiona's no-nonsense, down to earth attitude! She's tough but she's human too - always a nice mix!"
Christine Fieldhouse, National Journalist

"Working in the fashion industry we understand the pressure that people feel to stay slim and Fiona's advice has been vital to help the models on our books maintain their figures without jeopardising their health. In a world of endless "fad" diets Fiona's realistic weight loss techniques really are a breath of fresh air. Rather than promote denial and deprivation, Fiona offers practical and sensible advice for people with real life commitments that can't spend four hours a day in the gym and survive on a stick of celery for lunch!"
Neely Reyes - Founder, Sapphires Model Management

"Fiona's knowledge and approach to fat loss is second to none. Her approach is more about lifestyle changes and giving easy little tips to make a healthy, toned body that little bit easier...and the best thing is she practises what she preaches and is truly enthusiastic no matter how big or small your fat loss question is."
Lucy Miller, Fitness Editor, Health and Fitness Magazine

"Fiona Kirk knows what she's talking about and does so with passion and vivacity!" Holly Derry-Evans, Rude Health www.rudehealth.com

Table of Contents

Introduction

PART FIVE

Fat Burning Recipes

PART SIX

Introduction

Should we accept that the only way to shed fat for good is to change our eating habits for life and accept that it's going to be a slow, but ultimately healthy and successful process? Not necessarily. We can change some of our eating habits in just a few weeks if we really want to and see some great results that can motivate us into changing a few more.

Research shows that somewhere between 85% and 95% of dieters regain the weight they lost within five years and worse still, some end up heavier than when they started. But what about the 5-15% who reach their goal and maintain their initial weight loss? Surely they are the ones we all want to know about!

I decided the time had come to focus on the positives and embarked on a mission to find out what successful dieters do and why they not only lose the flab, but keep it off. After months of interviewing a great many people of both sexes and all ages, through a series of questionnaires, online forums, Facebook, Twitter and all manner of social networking methodology, I made a rather surprising discovery.

63% of the successful dieters found a *quick fix* diet that worked!

Initial fat loss spurred them into including some of the eating, drinking, exercise and lifestyle strategies they learned into their daily lives and not only did they reach their fat loss goal, but maintained it which illustrates that despite the negative press these kind of diets attract, they can work. And not just in the short term, but also in the long term.

This discovery led me to devour every diet book promising quick weight loss I could lay my hands on and scrutinise every research paper uncovering new and exciting ways to accelerate fat loss. This book is the result of my findings and presents a diet that results in maximum fat loss with maximum nourishment in minimum time and provides you with not only the knowledge to move closer to your goal but also the resolve to become one of the successful 5-15%. It is a short, punchy book which offers positive and workable recommendations, paying scant attention to the negatives that do little more than confuse and frustrate most dieters.

It is **not** a crash diet, it does **not** restrict calories or leave you short of nutritional goodness, it is **not** depressing, distressing, demotivating, demoralising or destructive and whilst it flags up the fat-gaining potential of regular consumption of certain carbohydrates it in **no** way fits into the *low carb* diet category.

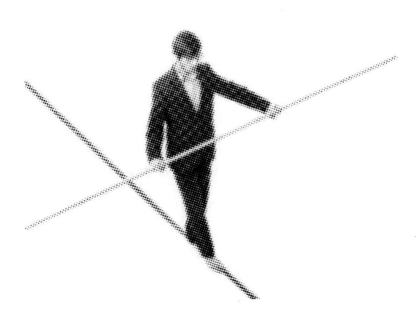

It is a balanced, energising, mood-boosting 14 day diet that brings together the latest research into faster fat loss (some proven, some just emerging but very exciting) coupled with some of the inspiring tips I learned from my *successful 63%* and focuses on:-

- foods that encourage fat loss
- foods that turn up the fat burning mechanism
- foods that delay hunger and conquer cravings
- foods that make us feel good
- foods that fire up our sex drive
- foods that help us sleep

It also reveals the latest research on exercise. When and how we exercise are just two of the critical elements to achieving maximum fat burning in minimum time and for most of us, time is precious and frustratingly short so adopting a strategy that ticks both boxes is vital.

Why does it work?
Women have around 34 billion fat cells and men have around 25 billion. When we gain fat we are not gaining new fat cells, we are merely expanding the ones we already have – think of a balloon gradually filling with water. They can become 5 to 6 times their size so to lose fat we have to get them to shrink and stay shrunk! There are certain nutrients, eating habits and lifestyle practices that can give them a proverbial *kick up the arse* and that's what we are going to concentrate on. Let the fat burning commence!

Note to readers

Those of you who have read my book *So What the F*** Should I Eat?* are aware that I included a 2 week diet plan for those occasions when time is tight and quick fat loss is vital. So, why am I offering another plan? Well, it's thanks to the vast numbers of you who contacted me to reveal that it worked and you were keen to continue. But, would it work long term? Could you make some alterations and still see weekly weight loss? Your enthusiasm encouraged me to get my *research hat* back on and find out more about why **rapid results in the early stages of a diet are crucial** and more importantly how we can build on initial success and avoid the often-inevitable loss of resolve that sees the pounds piling back on. You were my inspiration and the *2 Weeks in the Fast Lane* plan is the result. This diet is based on the original concept but now offers both **accelerated fat loss short term** and **continued fat loss long term**. A unique and exciting combination.

Part 1. Revelations

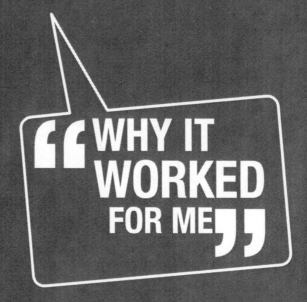

"Dairy products were major players in my breakfast, lunch, dinner and snack choices and boy were they packing on the pounds. Not any longer!"

The Aim

To find out what the 5-15% of successful dieters do in a bid to not only achieve their fat loss goal but also to maintain it long term.

The Plan

To devise a series of in-depth questions about diet, lifestyle, commitment, discipline, willpower, coping techniques, stumbling blocks, approach to exercise, knowledge about nutrition and a whole host of other stuff.

The Action

I invited dieters from all corners of the globe to respond/ communicate through as many channels as possible. Face to face, by means of my website/blog and other blogs, online forums and as many social networks as possible. I asked them to reveal **the 3 most important changes they made** ..... plus any other inspirational/unusual tactics employed.

The Results

The response was staggering and whilst I received a great many emails from failed dieters, indicating that positive and supportive help continues to be a major requirement in the weight loss game, I concentrated on the success stories and delved more deeply. 27% of the successful dieters revealed that they had indeed "finally accepted that the only way to shed fat for good was to change their eating habits for life" and had adopted a steady, healthy and successful fat loss lifestyle. They all get my total admiration (I would also encourage them to blog or write a book because some of their stories are quite extraordinarily inspiring).

However, what I truly didn't expect was that **a massive 63% of the successful dieters had found a *quick fix* 7-14 day diet that worked for them**. After months (sometimes years) of trial and error, involving all manner of diets (Atkins,

Weight Watchers, Blood Type, Cabbage Soup, Macrobiotic to name but a few), these dieters found a *quick fix* diet that was manageable, fitted in with their lifestyle, didn't involve foods or cooking methods they were unfamiliar with and the promised weight loss was achieved. They then used elements learned within the 7-14 days to not only continue to shed fat until they reached their goal but also to maintain their weight long term.

My Mission

I was onto something and I was excited! After years of believing much of what is reported about *quick fix* diets leading to long term weight gain and a whole host of other negatives it appears that this is not always the case. So I set about concentrating on the positive messages that some of these diets advocate, paying little attention to the emotionally-challenging overuse of words like *don't, avoid, restrict, refuse* and *quit* - a recipe for disaster for any dieter. I wanted to focus only on **why some of them can and do work**.

I am a nutritionist, not a psychologist and have modest academic knowledge about the underlying reasons as to why some people make diets work whilst others fail but what I do strongly believe is that permanent fat loss can only be achieved when we don't feel deprived, starving, miserable or negative. Food is fuel and regular fuelling is absolutely essential if we are to thrive; but food also provides a *feel good factor* that should never be trivialised. When we feel good, we focus and when we focus we move a lot closer to achieving our daily/lifetime goals. The *successful 63%* I chose to concentrate on inspired me not just because they reached their fat loss goals but also because they rubber-stamped my conviction that small changes to eating, drinking and lifestyle habits in the short term really can reap huge *feel good* rewards in the long term.

Here are just some of the discoveries they made which helped them to replace some of their *fat storing* habits with *fat busting* strategies and ultimately led to their success.

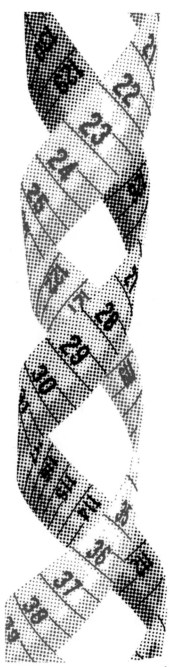

" I always had a can of Diet Coke nearby and believed that because it was diet it didn't add calories to my day. I learned that these supposedly negative calories did nothing to stem my dependence on sugar, replaced most of them with fresh fruit juices mixed 50/50 with sparkling water, regarded my love of Coca Cola as an occasional treat rather than a 4-a-day requirement and couldn't believe the reduction in my sugar cravings. I now understand that I was feeding my need for sugar which foiled every attempt at fat loss over many years."

" I love pasta and pasta loves me! It sits way too comfortably on my hips and thighs. I rarely dived into my favourite bolognese at lunchtime however; it was one of those after a hard day at the office regulars before settling down to watch a bit of telly before sloping off to bed. I learned that whilst I was enjoying the amazingly quick to prepare properties of this fabulous Italian export I was doing it at the wrong time of the day. Now, if I want pasta I have it at lunchtime when I know I need the immediate energy it provides to get me through the day but not at night when I am relishing a few hours of chill time but don't work it off and go to bed feeling bloated and stuffed ".

" I can't believe how much I now love fish! All those heads, bones and eyes staring up at me were enough to turn my stomach and whilst I watched others enjoying every bite, I just couldn't do it. But the diet I was trying to follow championed the importance of omega 3 fatty acids to stem my hunger pangs and for fat loss. I persevered and found a man behind the fish counter in my local supermarket whose enthusiasm and knowledge changed my life. He removed the head, bones and all the bits I couldn't cope with and presented me with not only the ready to cook fish but suggested ways to cook it. Now I eat fish at least 4 times a week."

"Despite having read, repeatedly over the years that breakfast is the most important meal of the day, I have always struggled to eat first thing in the morning. When I came across the Warrior Diet I was keen to have a go. To be honest, I didn't really understand much of what the author was talking about as there was so much science it made my head spin but, I didn't have to eat breakfast in order to lose weight so he had my attention! As long as I managed to drag myself out of bed and exercise first thing in the morning, I just had to refuel afterwards by eating small healthy snacks every couple of hours throughout the morning and it was not only manageable but worked for me. I lost 10lbs in the first week. I couldn't stick to the overly-stringent rules for more than a couple of weeks but I continued with the less is more in the morning approach and continued to lose weight. I no longer beat myself up because I can't eat very much early in the day, feel great and am slimmer than I have been in years"

" Loads of diets I have been on encourage me to write a food diary. At the end of every day you write down exactly what you have eaten and how much of it. This allows us to focus on where it is all going wrong. But I already know it is going wrong before I put pen to paper, so I lie. We all do! Yes, I mention the chocolate biscuit I may have had with my afternoon cup of tea, I just forget to mention that it wasn't just one, it was four! One diet that promised a loss of 8lbs in 8 days suggested that I bin the pen and paper and use my mobile phone to record everything I eat in a day in photo form then download it daily onto my computer to form a weekly diary. Revealing or what? I couldn't believe how much junk I managed to fit into a day. When it was right there in front of my eyes on the big screen I could see why I was fat and getting fatter - I was eating loads of food but not much of it was the kind of food that promotes weight loss. I followed the diet to the letter and within a couple of days I was loving the nightly big screen event - there was something empowering about looking at all those colourful health-giving foods that were now part of my day."

" It sounds ridiculous, but the reason I lost just over 3 stones and have maintained my weight loss is because I went on the Egg Diet! But, it wasn't because I followed the diet (well, I did for 5 days before I decided I never wanted to see another egg, ever again), it was because I learned how to steam food. Steamed vegetables are allowed occasionally, and as I had never steamed food before it was a completely new experience which has ultimately been a real life-changer. I bought a set of steam baskets, found lots of recipes on the internet about preparing really quick, healthy, tasty meals with the baskets and the frying pan has been relegated to the back of the cupboard."

"I know I am not alone when it comes to reaching the 5-a-day target and when I found a diet that suggested we should be aiming for more like 9-a-day (4 portions of fruit and 5 portions of vegetables!) I was tempted to put it back on the shelf. But, case studies reported between 7lbs and 12lbs lost in 2 weeks (plus health benefits) so I decided to give it a go. I stuck to the diet like a woman obsessed, lost loads of weight and had stacks of energy but boy, was I bored. I couldn't wait for the 2 weeks to be over. However, I realised that if I continued to eat this way most of the day, introducing other foods into my diet to make it more exciting I might be onto a winner. Fruits were fairly easy to include in my day but vegetables were still a struggle, so I focussed on the 5 vegetables that I really like and googled lots of different ways to prepare them (and had big portions to fill me up). I reached my target weight after 6 weeks and haven't put on a pound since and not only is my diet a lot more colourful but I have started experimenting with vegetables that I only ever regarded as hard work and my diet is anything but dull."

" I shared a flat with a Chinese girl who had a copy of an Asian Diet which she believed included all the foods and eating practices that had kept her nation fit and healthy for centuries (before western influences sneaked in). The first thing I noticed was that when we went shopping, almost no dairy products hit her trolley which made me realise just how much cows milk, butter and cheese were involved in my daily diet. She (and the book) introduced me to a few delicious alternatives, particularly nut and seed oils and butters and soya milk and when my weight started to plummet after only a week of making a few changes, I realised I had found the answer to my weight loss struggle. Continual consumption of dairy foods was not only packing on the pounds but also preventing me from kicking them into touch. I now eat the Asian way most days and whilst I still relish every bite of a take-away 4 Cheese Pizza it has become an occasional treat rather than a weekly must-have."

" I have always hated exercise and have tried every diet that involves phrases like ' bust fat without exercising'. Well if you have a phobia to exercise, why wouldn't you? Needless to say, I have never managed to maintain the weight loss that I have achieved in a couple of weeks for any longer than a couple of months. One quick fix diet I happened

upon whilst googling 'fast fat loss' reported that
'unlike any other form of exercise, rebounding
acts simultaneously on every single cell, muscle
and organ in the body. The results, when used
for even 2 or 3 minutes, 2 or 3 times a day, can
be amazing'. It also recommended watching TV
while I worked out and as I am continually
playing catch up with my favourite programmes I
reckoned it was worth a try. What can I say? I
became obsessed with that little trampoline and
instead of slobbing on the couch throughout
an entire movie, I started to bounce my way
through half of it! The diet also suggested that
I drank a large glass/small bottle of water after
each bouncing session and whilst I am still not
quite sure why the increased exercise and water
consumption combination works, I am living
proof that alongside a diet that includes lots
of healthy stuff but still allows me to have
good nights out with my friends, it does. After 6
months I am now very lean (body fat stabilised
at around 20%) and whilst I still hate exercise
and can think of nothing worse than forking out
my hard-earned cash on a gym membership, me and
my mini trampoline are not just flirting with each
other, we are in a long term relationship!"

" It seems that every diet I have ever attacked
involves way too much shopping. All the nutrients
that are important for fat loss appear to be
richest in fresh foods but after the first few
days of struggling to find the time to shop fresh

I lose the will to live and return to ready-made chilled foods that have a reasonable fridge life and can be on the table in super-quick time. But, this route has repeatedly foiled my attempts at fat loss. I imagine this is because they are often loaded with sugar, salt, fat or all three. But, when I spotted a diet on the internet that promised weight loss by eating foods from the freezer I was intrigued. I think it was featured in Good Housekeeping. All I had to do was load my trolley once a week with portion-controlled, calorie-counted meals, a few bags of frozen fruits and vegetables and I was good to go. By the end of 2 weeks I was 12lbs down and the rest of the family seemed happy enough with what appeared on the table. And, shopping time had been dramatically reduced. But, boredom soon set in. Same dishes, same tastes; it clearly wasn't going to work long term. However, what I learned was that frozen fruits and vegetables are packed with almost as much nutritional punch as their fresh counterparts (sometimes more) and if you have a few bags in the freezer you can create soups and smoothies quickly and that's what I focussed on - liquid nourishment! A fruit smoothie for breakfast (any spare going into a flask to be downed later in the day) and a nourishing soup for lunch or prior to my evening meal which seriously reduces how much I eat thereafter. I now always have at least six bags of frozen fruits and vegetables in the freezer and no longer have a weight problem."

" I went on a juice diet that promised I would lose 7lbs in 7 days and I did. Most of the juices were palatable, some were delicious and because I wasn't hungry I didn't stray too far from the plan but there was a lot of preparation involved which I knew was going to be a problem long term if I had any chance of continuing the weight loss. So, I decided to work out which of the juices really put the brakes on my cravings and kept my hunger at bay and found it was the ones which included flax seeds or flaxseed oil but sadly, they were the ones I loathed - way too oily and had to be forced down! A bit more reading made me realise that the good fats in flax played a big part in my weight loss because they filled me up and kept my blood sugar balanced for longer. But, surely I could get flax into my diet in other ways? I started sprinkling the seeds on my salads, drizzling the oil on my soups and vegetables and snacking on seed bars and nut and seed mixes that included them and I know for sure, now that I have lost over 2 stones that I have flax seeds to thank."

And here's my favourite...

"I read your book, So What the F*** Should I Eat?, followed your 2 week plan and guess what made the big difference? I binned the scales and used your Waistband Method. Instead of 'watching a little needle waver frustratingly from right to left' every morning as I had done with every diet I have ever been on, I put on a pair of trousers that were a size too small – everywhere! At the end of 2 weeks I could 'get a couple of thumbs between me and the waistband' as you promised and this really inspired me to keep going. I have always been a regular snacker as I was constantly hungry but instead of crisps and salty snacks which were my downfall, I started to keep a few of the healthy, filling snacks you suggest in my desk drawer – and still do. As you say, 'small changes can reap big rewards' and the fact that I now feel great in a pair of jeans I haven't been able to get over my hips for years is living proof."

Part 2. Fat Burning Foods

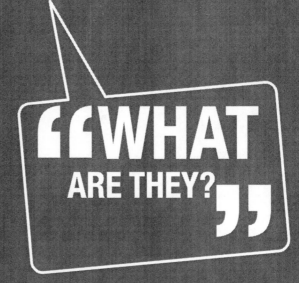

"WHAT ARE THEY?"

Astaxanthin, the 'magical' substance that gives salmon and its pink swimming companions their colour is truly earning its stripes as a fat loss warrior.

Calcium Is Not Just Good For Our Bones

Few are unaware of the importance of calcium in our diet to build and maintain strong bones and teeth but how much have you heard about its fat-busting properties? Recent research reveals that this *bone strengthener* may also be a *fat buster*.

A growing body of evidence indicates that a diet rich in calcium allows us to burn more calories per day. There is also some evidence that when calcium levels in the body are low the brain detects this and stimulates feelings of hunger, causing us to eat more. Conversely, medium to high levels send signals to the brain communicating that we are full, suppressing the desire to eat more.

Diets that include medium to high levels of calcium-rich foods have been found to result in up to half the amount of fat being stored to those providing low levels. This is believed to be as a direct result of calcium having the ability to reduce the action of a life-preserving enzyme system within the body which encourages fat storage.

- **LOW**   less than 600mg per day
- **MEDIUM**   600-1000mg per day
- **HIGH**   1000mg plus per day

It has also been suggested that increased calcium in the diet may reduce the transport of fat from the intestines into the bloodstream. The calcium binds with bile acids and increases the amount of fat we excrete through the bowel so instead of storing it we lose it! It has yet to be ascertained whether this process allows the body to determine between the fats we need and aid their absorption and those that lead to weight gain and ill-health. Fat is essential in our diet. If you read or hear otherwise, beware. It builds and repairs body cells, regulates hormones, helps us to absorb essential vitamins, combats cancer with its antioxidant properties, nourishes our skin and hair, buffers our nervous system and is a master source of energy. Some fats in our diet are only required in very small amounts but are important, others should be consumed daily, are vital to good health and efficient fat burning and should become our allies when we are trying to lose the flab. There is more to learn about these hard-working and supportive *fat loss friends* in the next section.

Many studies suggesting a possible link between achieving optimum calcium levels and weight loss concentrate on increasing our consumption of cow's milk products but from a nutritional point of view this may be a bit of a red herring. Milk is a valuable source of calcium up until about the age of 18 when we are still growing but thereafter we can have too much of a good thing. The protein in milk can acidify the blood and our bodies are forced to extract calcium from our bones to counteract this. Furthermore milk fat can contribute to inflammation within the body and possible intolerance to lactose, the sugar in milk products. Lactose intolerance is on the rise, chiefly because milk and its close cousins have become a staple in many diets. Milk with our morning cereals, milk in our coffee and tea, butter on our toast, cream in our cakes, cheese in our sandwiches and snacks, ice cream at the movies...the list goes on. To prevent this debilitating and difficult-to-manage condition whilst still reaping the calcium benefits, less is definitely more on the dairy front. The 2 Weeks in the Fast Lane plan achieves this by only including yoghurt, which because of its active *live* cultures actually improves lactose absorption and certain cheeses that fall into the low lactose category.

The bone remains of our earliest ancestors for whom dairy was a complete unknown (animals simply didn't hang around long enough to be milked) indicate that they ingested around twice as much calcium daily as we do now and they were lean - very lean. So what did they eat?

To build and maintain strong bones we need not only calcium but also magnesium, vitamin D, boron, manganese, molybdenum, vitamin K, zinc, copper, vitamin B6 and the Omega 3 and Omega 6 fatty acids. The diet of our early ancestors comprised of red meat and birds (and they ate every part of the animal including the organs), fish and shellfish (including the bones and heads which are very rich in calcium), root vegetables, sea vegetables, green leafy plants and birds' eggs (including the shells - another great source of calcium). This provided them with good levels of all of the above. And of course their active lifestyle further enhanced bone growth and kept them lean.

Whilst I am not advocating that you start crunching on eggshells and gnawing at bones, you will note that tinned salmon, sardines and anchovies feature regularly because they offer an ideal opportunity to get some calcium-rich bones into your day!

Increasing our consumption of cow's milk products to ensure good levels of calcium in our diet may be a bit of a red herring.

Calcium-rich foods included in the *2 Week Plan*

- *Total 0%* Greek yoghurt
- low fat natural cottage cheese
- regular tofu (smoked and unsmoked)
- silken tofu
- calcium-enriched soya milk
- parmesan cheese
- Swiss cheese 'with holes'
- goats' cheese cheddar
- ricotta cheese
- feta cheese
- fresh/frozen rhubarb
- fresh/frozen broccoli
- fresh/frozen spinach
- watercress
- bok choy
- kale
- dried/tinned beans
- tinned salmon
- fresh/tinned sardines
- fresh/tinned anchovies
- dried herbs
- edamame beans
- fresh nuts and their oils and butters
- fresh seeds and their oils and butters

OMG It's The Omega 3s

The phrase 'eating fat makes you fat' is so *old hat* now that it's somewhat embarrassing to recall that dieticians, nutritionists, the World Health Organisation and a host of other experts once deemed them to be everything that was bad for our health; amazingly, there are still a few who hold this view! Omega 3 essential fatty acids in particular are one of the great secrets to permanent fat loss and continue to be big news. They feed the furnace and aid fat loss by increasing metabolic rate and consequently energy production which is exactly the opposite of what happens when we cut calories. And, because of increased energy levels, we are more likely to be active and build muscle which further increases metabolic rate, helping to make fat loss permanent. They also taste great, make us feel fuller for longer, help to balance blood sugar levels, improve our mood and contribute to great skin, hair and nails. What's not to love?

Studies to date suggest some interesting theories:-

They help to maintain healthy blood sugar levels. It is vital that body cells are responsive to insulin, even the smallest amounts, to ensure an adequate uptake of glucose from the carbohydrates in our diet and amino acids from the protein to build muscle and minimise fat storage. Insulin receptors are found in cell membranes, the protective outer coating that controls what enters and exits a cell. When we add Omega 3s to our diet the membranes becomes more flexible, the receptors become increasingly sensitive to fluctuations and more responsive to the highs and lows in blood sugar levels, which are well-documented as contributors to weight gain and an increased risk of type 2 diabetes.

They inhibit the storage of calories as fat. It is important to remember that our species is programmed to survive and this involves storing energy as fat; an efficient source, as it provides 9kcals of energy per gram whereas carbohydrates and protein only provide 4kcals. This was vital to our ancestors as an insurance against times of starvation. A complex series of biochemical *saviours* within the body ensured that as much fat was stored as possible when food was available and metabolic rate slowed down to preserve energy stores when food was scarce. This process has been referred to as *catch-up fat after calorie restriction*.

Food is now plentiful and many of us eat what we want, when we want and these biochemical *saviours* have become the enemy in the fat loss game. They continue to store energy as fat for the lean times ahead totally unaware that these are unlikely to occur. This is why very low calorie diets invariably result in short term weight loss followed by fat gain. The *catch-up fat* mechanism moves into top gear!

A system of enzymes (catalysts that speed up chemical reactions) called *fatty acid synthase* is particularly proficient at storing calories as fat but there is growing interest in the role Omega 3s may have in reducing its power thus increasing the likelihood of fat being burned rather than

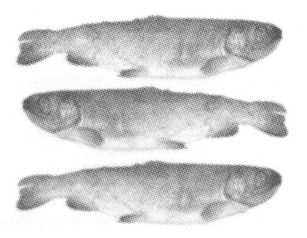

stored. In addition, studies suggest that they may be able to boost the production of certain enzymes involved in fatty acid oxidation which helps transport fats into the mitochondria (energy factories) of the cells for burning as energy.

They encourage glucose to be stored in muscle cells rather than fat cells. Omega-3s are involved in a phenomenon known as *fuel partitioning* - shifting the body from using fewer carbohydrates for fuel to using more fats as fuel. This is achieved by driving more of the sugars derived principally from the carbohydrates in our diet into muscle cells where it is temporarily stored in the form of glycogen. Glycogen is stored in both the liver and in muscle cells and is the first place the body turns to when we need quick energy between meals or when energy needs cannot be met by food intake alone, such as during intensive bouts of physical or mental activity. When glycogen stores run out, fat cells are forced to give up their energy stores and shrink in the process.

They increase thermogenesis. Thermogenesis is the production of heat by cells within the body. It creates a situation where the mitochondria in fat and muscle tissue produce heat instead of energy. Body temperature increases, creating a feeling of warmth, fat is used as fuel and calories are burned. Ongoing research suggests that Omega 3s may be able to directly influence genes that control how we store and burn fat. This may be due to a steroid-like substance in our bodies which, when bound to Omega 3s can *switch on* key genes involved in burning fat. Further research suggests that they may also *switch on* a protein which plays an important part in energy metabolism. This may result in more energy being dissipated as heat, increasing energy expenditure and decreasing stored fat.

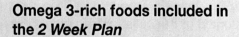

Omega 3-rich foods included in the *2 Week Plan*

- flax seeds (linseeds)
- flax seed oil
- walnuts
- walnut oil
- hemp seeds
- hemp seed oil
- fresh and smoked mackerel
- fresh and tinned sardines
- fresh and tinned anchovies
- rainbow trout
- fresh and tinned tuna
- dried and tinned kidney beans
- dried and tinned chickpeas
- avocado
- avocado oil
- fresh and frozen peas

If it's Fermentable it's Fat Burning!

There is great excitement all round regarding fermentable carbohydrates. They work within the body in such a way that they don't add much to our daily calorie intake, they promote bowel regularity, they reduce the chances of the pancreas getting over-tired in an effort to keep blood sugar levels constant and they are associated with less fat storage after a meal.

In essence, it's all about starch. The type of starch in carbohydrate foods predicts how quickly or slowly they are broken down into smaller and smaller glucose molecules by digestive enzymes in the mouth, the stomach and the small intestine before being absorbed into the bloodstream then delivered to the liver where they are either stored for later use or ferried off to body cells to create energy.

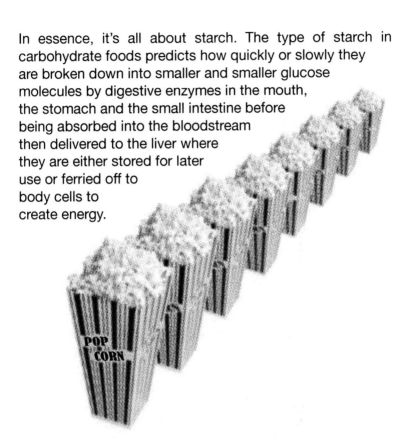

The starch in digestible carbohydrates is generally divided into two groups: rapidly digestible starch (digested within 20 minutes) and slowly digestible starch (digested somewhere between 20 minutes and 2 hours).

Rapidly digested starch (RDS) causes blood glucose to rise quickly, stay high for longer and drives up the production of insulin, which tells the body to make and store fat. RDS foods include potatoes and those made with white flour (bread and rolls, cakes, pastries, biscuits) plus many breakfast cereals.

Slowly digested starch (SDS) causes blood glucose to

rise less quickly, remain stable for longer, but still drives up the production of insulin, which tells the body to make and store fat, but not quite so swiftly. SDS foods include brown versions of most of the above. Principally because the nutrient-rich outer coating of whole grain foods has not been removed and therefore they take more chewing and are more slowly digested.

Non-digestible (fermentable) carbohydrates are a different breed and are so called because they contain **resistant starch (RS)**. They are largely resistant to the digestive process of being broken down into glucose molecules and absorbed through the gut wall into the bloodstream and just carry on down to the colon where they go through a fermentation process that produces short chain fatty acids (SCFAs) which have a number of health benefits:-

- They are protective of colon cells and associated with less genetic damage which can lead to cancer.
- They increase mineral absorption, particularly calcium and magnesium which are important for heart and bone health.
- By feeding the healthy bacteria, growth of unhealthy bacteria and their toxic by-products is suppressed.

Resistant starch has little effect on blood glucose levels, doesn't drive up the production of insulin which means the body is not encouraged to make and store fat.

Non-digestible carbohydrates have been shown to encourage fat loss in a number of ways:-

- They help to slow down the pace at which digestible carbohydrates get broken down thereby reducing the counter-productive blood sugar highs and lows which see us reaching for more starchy carbohydrates.

- They increase satiety - keeping us feeling fuller for longer so we eat less.
- They increase the absorption of calcium which is linked to reducing fat storage.
- They promote bowel regularity - constipation is no friend where fat loss is desired.
- They encourage a phenomenon known as *second meal effect* where the insulin response is controlled not just after a meal rich in fermentable carbohydrates but also for hours thereafter and well into our next meal resulting in less fat storage.

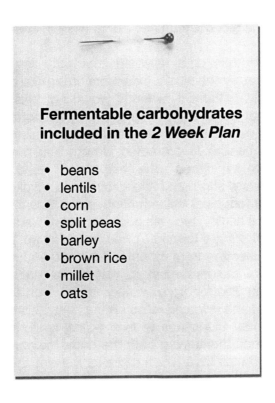

Fermentable carbohydrates included in the *2 Week Plan*

- beans
- lentils
- corn
- split peas
- barley
- brown rice
- millet
- oats

Spice up Your Diet

The notion that fat cells are simply a storage depot for body energy has now been irrefutably revised. Fat cells are actually very active and produce hormones that trigger metabolic processes in different parts of the body. The hormones produced include *oestradiol*, a precursor to *oestrogen* that controls reproduction, *leptin* which controls appetite by binding to receptors in the brain, telling us when we are full and *adiponectin* which controls blood sugar levels by heightening the body's sensitivity to *insulin*, the hormone that ensures the sugars absorbed from our diet are ferried out of the bloodstream and put to work to create energy.

Research has also revealed that fatty tissue produces inflammatory chemicals. Inflammation is a vital process within the body; without it, wounds would not heal and disease could not be reversed. It is the body's natural response to harmful substances where dead or dying tissue is disposed of and healing is promoted. **Acute** inflammation occurs when we are injured - the response is rapid, the duration is relatively short and the process is efficient. However, **chronic** (ongoing) inflammation is a different story. This is when the healing process goes into overdrive and damaging *free radicals* are formed. A *free radical* is an atom that has lost an electron from its outer orbit and becomes unstable and in a desperate bid to restore its stability randomly steals an electron from another atom which then becomes unstable and is forced to go on the hunt. This domino effect means that thousands of *free radical* reactions can occur in seconds threatening both the outer membranes of body cells and their DNA which can alter the way they behave.

When we overeat, fat cells expand and if they are regularly over-stuffed (particularly those around the midriff) inflammatory chemicals leap into action and interfere with the balance of the weight-controlling hormones. This can result in us becoming less sensitive to signals telling us we have had enough to eat so we eat more and our insulin response is dulled, creating increased episodes of hypoglycaemia (low blood sugar) which prompts us to reach for more food to counteract the tiredness, fuzzy brain, irritability and low mood that go with the territory.

Dieters often blame the desire to eat more on a lack of willpower and whilst desire plays a huge part in what, when and how much we eat, our biochemistry has a lot to answer for. The body will always do the very best it possibly can to ensure that homeostasis (balance) is maintained. Survival is its number one priority and no matter how often or seriously the balance is disrupted, it will continue to make adjustments to try to get things back on track.

Ballooning fat cells caused by overeating are not the only reason the inflammatory chemicals are stimulated and the healing process is forced into overdrive. Another major cause is what we actually eat. The altered fats found in fried, fast, processed and junk foods and foods with crazy levels of added sugars which invade most Western diets (and increasingly, global diets) are the chief culprits here. But let's focus on the foods that minimise the likelihood of inflammation and enable the weight-controlling hormones to do what they do best; control our appetite and encourage efficient blood sugar management. These include fruits, vegetables, oily fish, nuts and seeds and their oils, whole grains and herbs and spices.

Herbs and spices are important because they are very rich in antioxidants, substances that protect body cells from the damage created when the inflammatory process is in full swing. Antioxidants are like protective parents that form a shield around our body cells and absorb *free radicals* which are neutralised, lose their destructive energy and are safely excreted from the body. If you cut an apple in half and leave one half uncovered for 20 minutes you can see *free radical* damage occurring. The apple starts to go brown and dries up because it reacts with the oxygen in the air causing *free radicals* to be formed. If you soak the other half in lemon juice however, it retains its creamy, white colour and texture. This is because it has been protected by the vitamin C in lemon juice. Vitamin C is a powerful antioxidant.

The antioxidant-rich, anti-inflammatory properties of herbs and spices encourage fat burning whilst reducing fat storage. They also add flavour and excitement to food which results in reduced salt consumption. Too much salt prompts fluid retention, another fat loss adversary.

But, what about the supposed metabolism-boosting attributes of herbs and spices? The possibility that there may be foods that can achieve this and encourage more fat to be used for fuel is tantalising not only to scientists but also to dieters. Thus far results are confusing and contradictory. When we have just eaten, our body temperature automatically rises as energy is created to metabolise the food but it's not significant. Despite the lengthy lists we may come across of 'foods guaranteed to boost metabolism', there is actually only one substance that has proven itself to be a real thermogen and that's *capsiate* which is found in chillies but sadly we have to eat rather a lot of them to get the thermogenic effect and because most chillies are much richer in *capsaicin*, the substance that gives them their intense heat this may present a few problems for many of us! However, scientists have created a new variety of sweet pepper called CH-19 which doesn't contain *capsaicin* but is rich in *capsiate*. We could see these taking centre stage in the vegetable section fairly soon so look out for them.

Herbs and spices included in the *2 Week Plan*

- chilli
- garlic
- turmeric
- cayenne
- black pepper
- cinnamon
- cumin
- mint
- mustard
- oregano
- parsley
- rosemary
- thyme
- ginger

The Power of Pink

The pigment responsible for giving salmon, prawns, langoustine, lobster and their pink swimming companions their colour is a carotenoid called *astaxanthin* which is synthesised as a direct result of the microalgae they feed on. Research suggests that this naturally-occurring plant chemical may be the most powerful antioxidant to go under the microscope thus far and has been shown to provide the body with an internal sunscreen, protecting us from the damaging effects of UV rays from the sun. Small amounts of UV light are beneficial as it enables the body to make Vitamin D which aids in the absorption of calcium, helping to form and maintain strong bones but few are unaware that over-exposure contributes to prematurely ageing skin and in some cases skin cancer. This exciting discovery has already led to astaxanthin being included in anti-ageing skin care products and sunscreens.

Furthermore, because astaxanthin has been proven to cross the blood–brain barrier, it offers protection to the brain, the central nervous system and the eyes.

It has also been shown to increase the usage of fat as an energy source and accelerate fat burning during exercise. A group of Japanese researchers recently demonstrated that mice given astaxanthin along with a high fat diet had significantly lower body weight and body fat levels compared to mice fed on a high fat diet of a similar calorie count. In another study, mice were given astaxanthin along with a daily exercise routine. After four weeks the animals were placed on a treadmill to test a range of physical parameters and similar to the study above, astaxanthin increased fat usage during exercise. At present, no human studies have been concluded but researchers are confident that this powerful *pink* substance may play an important role in the fight against our globally-increasing waistlines.

There is another reason why astaxanthin is a valuable addition to a diet focussed on fat loss; its anti-inflammatory properties. As discussed in the last section, inflammation is no friend where fat loss is the goal and it is antaxanthin's role in good gastric health that is important here. Inflammation in the 21st century gut is on the increase and a condition known as *leaky gut syndrome* is largely to blame.

The digestive tract consists of a long tube, which connects the mouth to the anus. After food is swallowed it passes through the oesophagus to the stomach, where it is churned up with acid and broken down into tiny particles by stomach enzymes. These then pass into the small intestine which is around 20 feet long and its major function is to digest and absorb the valuable nutrients from the food particles that arrive from the stomach before releasing them into the bloodstream. Then it's off to the liver for further processing to produce the *essentials* which are quickly delivered to body cells to provide the energy to make new cells, repair cells that are worn out and generally keep us in good health.

The inner lining of the small intestine can, however become inflamed due to infection, because of toxic substances within foods or as a result of the over-consumption of processed fats, sugars and food additives, which over time weaken its permeability. When the gut becomes *leaky*, overly-large and damaging food molecules enter the bloodstream causing an immediate response by the immune system which recognises these invaders as a threat to health. As they pass through the liver they have to be detoxified to limit the potential damage but this places an enormous burden on the liver, stressing its detoxification capability and resulting in these substances being only partially processed and allowed to build up. In a bid to restore its health and efficiency and prevent these partially-processed toxins from being released back into the bloodstream, the liver is forced to pack them up and send them off for safe storage and our fat cells are only too willing to accommodate! Frustratingly, it is hard enough to encourage fat cells to release their energy and shrink because they are programmed to store fat for survival but it is even harder when they are storing toxins which when released into the bloodstream are likely to create havoc and compromise our health. This is damage limitation at its best but can be a major stumbling block when we want to shift fat.

Fat loss becomes a whole lot easier, quicker and maintainable in the long term when the cells that line the small intestine are healthy and strong. Astaxanthin has not only shown itself to be protective of the outer membranes of these cells, reducing the chance of toxic substances compromising their permeability but also has the ability to mount a massive anti-inflammatory effect should toxic substances sneak through into the bloodstream. This is clearly a substance that is earning its stripes as a fat loss warrior.

'Pink' Foods included in the *2 Week Plan*

- salmon
- shrimps
- prawns
- crayfish
- crab
- lobster
- rainbow trout
- red caviar

Fork Your Way to Feeling Good

Dopamine is a neurotransmitter that helps control the brain's reward and pleasure centre and the chemical messages it communicates to the brain regulate emotional responses to enable us not only to seek reward but also to take action to move towards it. Depriving ourselves of foods that give us pleasure is perhaps one of the most documented reasons dieters give up after relatively short periods. If we don't feed our desires, we wither. Whether it's food, love, attention or praise, we all need rewards in some shape or form and food definitely has the ability to give us a *culinary hug* when the chips are down. But to ensure we don't reach for the *Häagen-Dazs* and wolf down an entire tub in one sitting, we have to focus on foods that encourage a drip-feed effect.

Several studies indicate that people who are overweight or obese produce low levels of dopamine so are unconsciously driven to seek out ways to raise the level with food to get the *feel good factor* back. The quickest way to restore levels is by eating foods that release their sugars rapidly but these foods invariably lead to further weight gain. Worse still, repeated consumption desensitises the receptors in the brain which means more of the same is required to get the reward we seek.

Happily, there are other ways to increase dopamine levels naturally. One is through exercise. Among the early changes seen when individuals engage in an aerobic training program are mood elevation, heightened energy levels, enhanced self-confidence and self-esteem, lower anxiety levels, resistance to depression and improved coping ability. Higher levels of dopamine have been recorded following aerobic exercise training in several studies and there is also evidence that levels remain elevated for longer. Interestingly, improvements in the physical capabilities and mood of Parkinson's disease patients have been recorded following six to eight weeks of aerobic walking training. Dopamine levels are commonly low in people with Parkinson's disease. It has yet to be ascertained whether certain types of aerobic exercise achieve higher levels than others or indeed whether levels stay elevated for longer dependent on the time of day we exercise but one relatively small study suggests that 30 minutes of jogging first thing in the morning on an empty stomach may have the edge. Further research is ongoing which may provide a clearer picture but findings so far present yet another good reason to *get physical* on a daily basis.

The brain cells which manufacture dopamine use *phenylalanine* as the raw material. Phenylalanine is an essential amino acid found in the brain and blood plasma that can convert in the body to *tyrosine*, another amino acid which in turn is used to synthesise dopamine. Amino acids are building blocks of protein so to encourage good levels of

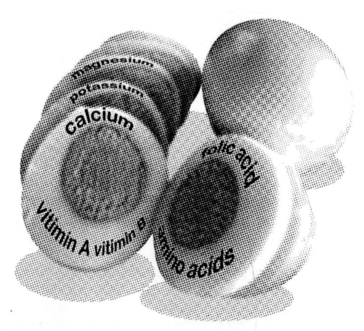

dopamine, we need to eat protein foods, particularly those rich in phenylalanine and tyrosine. We also need good levels of certain vitamins and minerals which feed the enzymes (catalysts) which promote the production of dopamine. Iron, copper, folic acid, and vitamins B3, B6 and C are the important ones, all of which are supplied in good amounts in the 2 Week Plan.

Foods that boost dopamine production included in the *2 Week Plan*

- fish
- shellfish
- chicken
- turkey
- venison
- eggs
- oats
- bananas
- peanuts
- pumpkin seeds
- sesame seeds
- lentils
- chickpeas

Part 3. Fat Burning Boosters

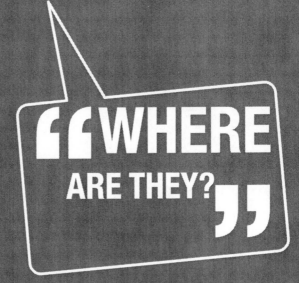

Sex in not only a great de-stressor but burns up around 6-7kcals per minute. Fat burning, physically demanding and fun; what's not to love?

Alcohol and Caffeine - Not As Bad As You May Think!

Alcohol

There is evidence that consumption of two to four glasses of red wine a day reduces the risk of a heart attack by up to an astonishing 32% due to the protective combination of the alcohol and *resveratrol* (and a few other plant chemicals therein). Music to the ears of all who are partial to the occasional glass or two! So, can the odd tipple feature in a fat loss diet? In some cases, yes. It has a lot to do with what we drink, when we drink, how much we drink and what we eat before, during and after a glass of our favourite *poison*!

There are two very important points to stress here. One is that if you don't currently drink alcohol, don't for heavens' sake take it up in a bid to cut your risk of heart disease - a healthy diet and lifestyle will take care of that (same applies to infrequent drinkers). Secondly, if you are a heavy drinker or alcohol plays a major part in your life, you are at risk of potentially serious health problems so you should make every effort to get consumption under control.

However, people who drink moderately (max 2 units per day for men, 1 unit for women) and are able to control their consumption (spread over the week as opposed to bingeing at the weekend) and don't have any of the absolute reasons why we shouldn't be drinking alcohol (pregnancy, on medication, operating heavy machinery, poor health history etc) can take comfort in the fact while they are enjoying some down-time with glass in hand, there may be a few benefits!

Its heart-friendly properties are not the only benefit. A number of studies have found that adults with moderate alcohol intakes are at significantly lower risk of developing type 2 diabetes than adults who don't partake and analysis

of some 15 studies concluded that moderate consumpti
reduces the risk by around 30%. It has been suggested th
this may be associated with improved insulin sensitivity. B
what is insulin sensitivity and why is it so important for f
loss?

When the incredibly efficient mechanism that ensures th
glucose derived from what we eat and drink is prevente
from rising too high or dropping too low in the bloodstrea
it's all good, the glucose gets ferried off to feed our insatiab
brain cells, then on to the trillions of other body cells to creat
energy as required. But, if this mechanism is put under stres

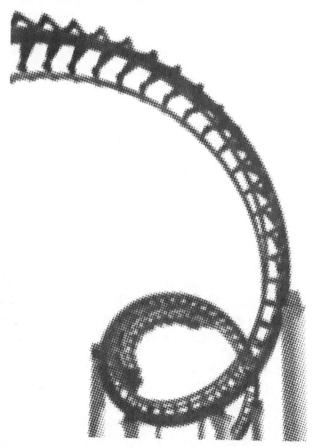

because we insist on pouring glucose into the bloodstream at an accelerated pace through our consumption of foods that require very little processing (sugary cereals, cakes, biscuits, pastries, alcohol, fizzy drinks and the rest...) it considers throwing in the towel and demanding time out.

The pancreas, which has the unenviable task of keeping glucose in the bloodstream within safe limits gets over-worked, the body cells which gobble up glucose for energy when it's needed tire of opening the gates to let yet more glucose in and the whole system becomes less efficient. So, if the glucose continues to pour into the bloodstream and the body is programmed to keep things in balance how does the system cope? Ultimately it doesn't. Either the pancreas produces less and less insulin and type 2 diabetes develops or the body cells take in less and less glucose, causing abnormally high levels of insulin in the blood (hyperinsulinemia) which can lead to high blood pressure, high levels of damaging cholesterol and heart disease. Both scenarios are to be avoided not just because of the debilitating health issues but also because of the well-documented link both conditions now have with obesity.

So, how can you reap a few health benefits and enjoy the odd glass whilst following a fat loss program? Best advice is to have a glass of good red wine with your evening meal and only occasionally have another (Cabernet Sauvignon, Pinot Noir and Merlot are richest in protective flavonoids). If your social life involves dining out, meeting friends/colleagues for a drink or entertaining at home, here are a few tips that can minimise the addition of calories without meaning you have to say "no" to invitations:-

- Alcohol raises blood sugar very quickly, so always have a protein-rich snack before or with a drink (a couple of oatcakes with nut butter, a small pot of *live* natural yoghurt with fresh fruit, a chicken leg, a cold boiled egg, some crunchy baby vegetables with a small pot of hummus, a handful of almonds) to moderate the sugar spike.
- Alcohol dehydrates, so for every drink you have, have two large glasses of water; you will have to go to the ladies/mens room more often but you will seriously cut down on the amount of alcohol you consume. And, have a few glasses of water before bed (and keep another one by the bed) to help re-hydrate and ensure you feel fresh the next morning.
- Alcohol increases your appetite, lessens your resolve and removes inhibitions (!!!) so always make sure you have a friend/partner around to keep you on track.
- Avoid fizzy mixers at all costs – they are full of sugar and the *diet* alternatives are no better, they just increase your desire for more sugar and consequently more alcohol.
- Avoid all *lite* beers, *alcopops* and ready-mixed, spirit-based cocktails – sugar, sugar and yet more sugar!
- Aim for good quality wine, spirits *on the rocks* or with natural unsweetened fruit juice.
- Cocktails can be dangerous and often high in sugar, but if you stick to *Breezes, Martinis, Sours, Manhattans, Screwdrivers, Punches* and *Pimms* (no sugar added, just the sweetness from the fruit), you shouldn't get into too much trouble. And, don't forget the highly nutritious, satisfying and delicious Bloody Mary or Bloody Caesar.
- Mix white wine with soda water to make it last twice as long and half the calories. If you can't bear to dilute it, opt for dry whites as these contain fewer calories than sweeter wines.
- Follow in the footsteps of celebrities and enjoy a glass

of *bubbly* if funds allow. In general you drink less as it's served in smaller glasses and the bubbles fill you up.

- Most measures of spirits poured at home are larger than those served in bars and pubs with the result that your drink will probably contain twice as many calories. If you do a lot of entertaining at home, it's worth investing in a spirits measure. Also, always pour spirits into the glass before adding ice or mixers, so you can actually see just how much alcohol is involved.

- Steer clear of beer, lager and cider as they're loaded with calories. And the higher the alcohol content, the more calories they contain. For example, a pint of standard beer contains around 160 calories, whereas a bottle of strong lager can contain more like 220 calories.

- Beware of trendy wine bars. Many serve spirits in double measures as the standard, with the result that you get double the calories. Some pubs also serve 35ml measures of spirits rather than 25ml measures and so also contain more calories. Finally, watch out for huge wine glasses – some are so large that a glass of wine may actually be close to a third of a bottle.

- Avoid creamy liqueurs after dinner and instead have a single shot of brandy if you really fancy ending your meal in style. Most cream-based liqueurs contain around 80-100 calories per 25ml measure compared with 50 calories in a single brandy.

- Remember that *happy hours* are designed to get you to drink more and keep you in the same place all night. Unfortunately, this means while the bar gains pounds, so do you as you indulge in far more drinks than you normally would.

- Why not offer to drive from time to time so that you won't be able to drink anything other than fresh fruit and vegetable juices, sparkling water or soda and lime!

Caffeine

It's hard to find anyone who can bin the cappuccino habit long term, but there is evidence that it may not be the devil it is believed to be from a fat loss point of view. Bodybuilders and athletes have been using caffeine to reduce body fat for over 20 years but it is only recently that its fat-burning properties have been further investigated. As with alcohol, it's all about the what, the when and the how.

Properly used, caffeine stimulates the central nervous system, increases the use of body fat as fuel and preserves glycogen levels (the glucose stored in the liver and muscles). But it is also a diuretic so it promotes the loss of water from our body cells and raises body temperature, so we overheat. Studies focussed on professional athletes reveal that caffeine taken 3 hours prior to testing allow them to perform both longer and harder before exhaustion and increase the use of fat for fuel, thereby sparing the glycogen stored in their muscles which, when depleted causes what is commonly known as *hitting the wall* where energy levels take a major dive and more glucose-rich foods and drinks have to be consumed to enable them to continue.

But, few of us are professional athletes so can caffeine play a role in fat burning for the slightly less physical amongst us? Yes. Caffeine increases the number of calories the body burns at rest. A single 100mg dose of caffeine can increase our metabolic rate by 3-4% for at least an hour and a half afterwards. 100mg consumed every two hours for 12 hours has also been shown to increase our daily metabolic rate by 8-11% (one cup of reasonably strong coffee contains anywhere between 65mg and 115mg of caffeine). However, it doesn't have the same effect in everyone. The rise in the metabolic rate is around 150 calories in lean individuals, but only around 80 calories if we are overweight.

One study compared the effects of caffeine in 10 lean and

10 obese women. The rise in metabolic rate following the consumption of caffeine was just under 5% in the obese women and just over 7% in the lean women and although the effects of the caffeine on the metabolic rate could no longer be seen the following day, both groups were still burning between 10% and 30% more fat at rest than before the caffeine trial.

Now, I am not encouraging a cup of coffee every 2 hours over a 12 hour period! Coffee has rather many downsides:-

- Many of the chemicals in coffee irritate the stomach lining causing an increase in stomach acid leading to digestive disorders.
- It raises blood pressure.
- It decreases quality of sleep.
- It causes problems with blood sugar control.
- It excites more rapid peristaltic movements of the intestines resulting in shortened transit times and less absorption of nutrients.
- It leaches calcium from the bones increasing the risk of osteoporosis.
- It is one of most heavily pesticide-sprayed crops.

However, caffeine does have a role to play in fat loss. When used in conjunction with a healthy lifestyle it can make losing fat a little faster and a little easier, particularly when consumed before exercise.

So if you are a *coffee-head* here's the plan. Have a double espresso or a small cup of strong filtered coffee first thing in the morning, get out for a brisk walk, jog or run for 30 minutes, have at least one large glass of water when you get back home, shower and dress then have a fruit-rich breakfast before or on the way to work and try substituting your morning coffee with a cup of green tea which is a rich source of caffeine but doesn't pose the health risks of coffee mentioned above AND doesn't involve milk which can hinder fat loss or sugar which only adds calories to your day. And, whatever you do, don't resort to caffeinated fizzy drinks like *Coca Cola* or *Red Bull* in a bid to boost your caffeine levels and increase fat burning; there are around 8 spoonfuls of sugar in every can!

Make Your Brown Fat Cells Work for You

Most body fat is white fat, the bulky stuff that stores excess calories, makes up cell membranes, insulates nerve cells, cushions our organs and sits on our hips. But we also have small amounts of brown fat and brown fat cells not only have a much richer blood supply but are jam-packed with mitochondria, the energy powerhouses. That makes them a great deal more metabolically active and instead of making energy, they make heat using fat and glucose from the bloodstream for fuel. This means that basal metabolic rate (BMR) increases and more calories are burned. Some studies estimate that active brown cells can burn up as much as 20% of our daily calorie intake. We are born with a good supply and as babies we have the ability to turn white fat cells into brown fat cells to keep the body warm but sadly, as we age the process becomes less efficient. However, there is growing evidence that adults retain some brown fat and when we are exposed to cold they become more metabolically active and burn more fat. Taking cold baths and showers, swimming in the cold waters of our British shores or unheated swimming pools, exercising on winter mornings in skimpy shorts and a T-shirt or wearing specially designed clothing that keep the areas that are rich in brown fat cells cool (the armpits and the neck area) have all been investigated. Some of these methods are fairly extreme so unless your health is good, you are advised to consult your doctor before giving them a try.

Other ways of encouraging brown fat cell activity and prompting increased calorie burning to keep the body warm may be to turn down the heating thermostat, wear fewer clothes and sleep in a cool room. If you are over 50 you may remember when the heating only went on in the dead of winter and you always slept in a cold room with the window open - that's when most people were slim so there may be something in it! Read the research to date on brown fat - it's fascinating stuff and could hold the key to increased fat burning in the future.

Sex, Sleep and Sunshine - Let's Have More of These!

Sex

Anti-ageing researchers have proposed that people showing the slowest ageing rates often have a particularly well-developed libido and sex life. The main libido-determining hormone is *testosterone* and whilst women don't want this sex hormone to dominate (who of us girls want a moustache?), men don't want it to underachieve, so healthy levels are the goal for both sexes. An added bonus is that this hormone is a fat burner when certain vitamins and minerals are supplied through our diet so it's not just about eating more oysters!

Like a car, fat cells have brakes and accelerators. The parts of a fat cell that accelerate the release of fat are called *beta receptors*, while the parts of a fat cell that put the brakes on fat loss are known as *alpha receptors*. Beta receptors help fat loss because they increase the rate at which stored fat is broken down as well as increasing blood flow in fat tissue. In contrast, alpha receptors hinder fat loss, slowing the flow of fat out of the cells. The distribution of these brakes and accelerators explains, to a degree why we lose body fat faster in certain parts of the body than in others.

If a fat cell has more beta receptors, it releases stored fat more quickly and this is where testosterone appears to help. Testosterone can increase the number of receptors, making it easier to lose stored fat. It has also been shown to limit the storage of fat; when fat cells are exposed to testosterone in a test tube, the activity of the enzyme system that promotes fat storage, *fatty acid synthase* is dramatically reduced.

Foods that Boost/Balance Testosterone levels in the *2 Week Plan*

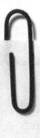

- apples
- broccoli
- red peppers
- chickpeas
- garlic and onions
- peanuts
- green leafy vegetables
- olives
- eggs
- lean beef

Sleep

A number of studies have found that those who get less than 6 hours of sleep per night tend to gain more weight over time than people who get 7 to 8 hours. The production of two hormones, *leptin* and *grehlin* which control hunger and fullness are influenced by how much or how little sleep we get. Leptin controls appetite, is produced by the fat cells and tells the brain when energy stores are replenished and we have had enough to eat. Grehlin controls hunger, is produced in the stomach and tells the brain when we are hungry and need nourishment. When these hormones are working optimally we are better able to control when we eat and how much we eat but unfortunately they are easily disrupted. If the signals to the brain are scrambled it is all too easy to just go along with our desires resulting in us gorging rather than grazing and likely weight gain.

Leptin levels peak when we are asleep so if we don't get enough sleep levels drop and if we are regularly deprived, they stay depressed and the brain interprets this as a reduction in energy stores prompting us to eat more in an effort to get the balance back. Continued lack of sleep also causes grehlin levels to rise, which means our appetite is repeatedly stimulated and we want more food. The two combined set the stage for overeating so clearly, getting our 8 hours a night is critical. But, what if you are one of the millions for whom a good nights' sleep is the goal but rarely a reality? You either can't get to sleep and toss and turn for hours or you wake up in the wee small hours and can't get back to sleep so you end up doing the ironing or checking your emails at five in the morning; your leptin and grehlin levels are all over the place and fat loss isn't going to be easy, so what can you do?

Have a bedtime snack that includes foods that encourage the production of the sleep-inducing neurotransmitter *serotonin*. When you are trying to shift fat, the suggestion that you should eat before you *hit the sack* sits uncomfortably with most but when you understand that sleep deprivation promotes weight gain and balanced blood sugar levels and a good nights' sleep aid weight loss you may want to reconsider.

Our serotonin levels are directly related to the amount of *tryptophan* (an essential amino acid found in protein foods) in the blood and as blood and brain levels of tryptophan rise and fall, so do levels of serotonin. Tryptophan can be the *runt of the litter* when it comes to competing with the other amino acids to get from the bloodstream into the brain, but a little carbohydrate added to a protein-rich snack creates a diversion allowing tryptophan to take the main stage.

Foods that Boost Serotonin levels in the *2 Week Plan*

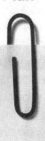

- soya milk
- yoghurt
- cottage cheese
- turkey
- bananas
- peanuts
- oats
- rye
- lettuce
- dark chocolate
- lemon juice

Sunshine

Vitamin D, which is essential for the absorption of calcium into our bones to keep them strong is produced within the body when we are exposed to sunlight but recent research reveals that many of us are deficient in this vitamin. Further research indicates that women who are D-deficient carry between 40% and 80% more abdominal fat than their D-rich counterparts. Now is definitely the time to become D-aware! As previously discussed, fat cells are not just storage depots; they are metabolically active and vitamin D, which is stored in fat cells has an important role to play in regulating how much fat we store and how much we burn. We know that leptin, the hormone that controls appetite is produced by the fat cells and tells the brain when energy stores are replenished and we have had enough to eat but like sleep deficiency, it appears that vitamin D deficiency can interfere with this appetite-suppressing hormone causing us to eat more.

Because vitamin D is stored in fat cells, one would imagine that the bigger our fat cells, the more vitamin D we are able to store, allowing its release into the bloodstream for bone building and cellular health but quite the opposite has been noted. The fatter we are, the higher our risk of deficiency because vitamin D gets *locked* inside fat cells and unavailable for use. In one study, a group of obese adults (BMI above 30) and a group of lean adults (BMI of 19-24) were exposed to the same amount of UVB rays and blood levels of vitamin D in the lean adults rose by almost double those in their obese counterparts, indicating that when we are overweight we need a lot more.

Vitamin D deficiency has also been shown to disrupt the delicate balance of insulin production by the pancreas and increase the possibility of insulin resistance which over time leads not only to weight gain but also an increased risk of type 2 diabetes.

Vitamin D is primarily synthesised in the skin after exposure to sunshine. It was previously thought that as little as 5-10 minutes of sun exposure on arms, legs and face three times a week without sunscreen between 11am and 2pm during the spring, summer and autumn should provide a light-skinned individual with adequate vitamin D and allow for some storage of any excess for use during the winter with minimal risk of skin damage. Those with dark skin may require twice or three times the exposure. However, a recent survey in the UK indicates that more than half of the adult population are deficient in vitamin D and in the winter about 1 in 6 people show a severe deficiency. If the body cannot produce enough vitamin D because of insufficient sunlight exposure, we need to up our levels with D-rich foods but even then we may be short.

A new report has found that a minimum of 4000IU of vitamin D is required daily to maintain optimal blood levels. Around 3500 men and women had their vitamin D levels measured and completed online surveys to monitor vitamin D status and health outcomes over five years. The aim of this study was to assess how much vitamin D is needed to ensure optimal rather than just adequate levels in the average person.

The researchers found that daily intakes of between 4000IU and 8000IU are needed to maintain blood levels of vitamin D to effectively reduce the risk of diseases such as breast cancer, colon cancer, multiple sclerosis and type 1 diabetes and importantly they also found that this dose was very safe.

So, from a health and fat loss point of view, daily exposure of your skin to sunlight and a diet packed with foods rich in vitamin D are crucial. You may also wish to have your vitamin D levels checked. A simple blood test available at your GP's surgery measures the level of a chemical called *25 hydroxy-vitamin D*, the chemical formed in the liver during the process that converts sunlight into vitamin D and if the sunshine and the D-rich foods don't see you reaching the mark, supplementation may be required.

Vitamin D-rich Foods in the *2 Week Plan*

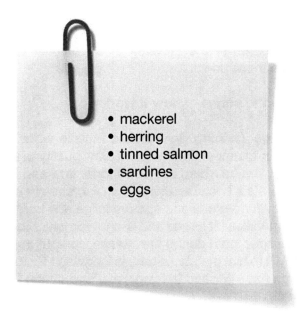

- mackerel
- herring
- tinned salmon
- sardines
- eggs

Exercise for Fat Burning - The Latest News...

This is predominantly a book about getting the nutritional edge and understanding how, when and why the foods we consume can either add to our waistlines or reduce them, but it would in no way be complete if the deserved respect was not shown to those who work tirelessly to augment our understanding of the most up to date methods of busting fat with the aid of regular exercise. They know we don't want to spend hours in the gym doing the same old routine, they also appreciate that we are probably short of time and total dedication is tough. As with nutrition, confusion reigns but there are a few themes emerging which you may wish to consider if you are seriously committed to building muscle to bust fat.

If you want to see great and long-lasting results from the following well-researched exercise combination to find the fit, lean and toned body you know is lurking somewhere under those excess pounds of flesh, you may wish to delve more deeply into the science. If so, read some of the many studies available, buy a book that covers this type of programme in detail or enlist the services of a personal trainer who practices these principles.

Here are the bones of how it works:-

Resistance Training. To increase muscle whilst shedding body fat in the most time-efficient way, quality over quantity is the key. You train hard but for a shorter time and fat burning is accelerated because there is an increased secretion of both *growth hormone* and *noradrenaline*, the hormones that help to mobilise fat stores and use fat for fuel. More calories are expended both during the intense workout and because your BMR (basal metabolic rate) is increased for many hours after you have finished training - that's when the fat burning kicks in.

By using dumbbells, exercise machines, your own body weight, bottles of water, elastic tubing, ankle and wrist weights or exercise bricks, muscles are strengthened by pitting each group against a force (resistance). To develop a muscle you must work all the fibres within it which means pushing them to their limit for short periods of time, resting them briefly then repeating the process. You work with a weight that is heavy enough so that the last few repetitions become difficult to perform. This is not the kind of exercise where you chat to a friend while you work out. It requires concentration and determination. When a muscle is overloaded, lactic acid is produced causing the *burn* in the muscle that ultimately leads to muscular fatigue – you have to push past that sensation and ensure your mind doesn't give up before your body. The rest between repetitions enables the lactic acid to be flushed from the bloodstream, allowing the muscles to be refreshed before working them again.

Recommendations vary but generally 30-40 minutes, three times a week is a good goal. To allow the muscles to repair and regenerate 48hrs should be allowed between sessions. This enables protein synthesis to take place (the process by which the body repairs muscle tissue) preventing injury.

And it's never too late to start. In one study of elderly men and women (average age 87) who lifted weights three times a week for ten weeks, muscle strength increased by a staggering 113% on average. This improvement in strength enabled them to walk 12% faster than before, climb 28% more stairs and lose excess body fat.

Interval Training. Whilst resistance training is the most effective for fat burning for many hours after a workout, it should be coupled with aerobic exercise for a number of reasons. The cardiovascular system becomes more efficient at delivering oxygen to working muscle, delaying the lactic acid build-up which allows you to train at a higher level of intensity. Aerobic exercise also expands the network of blood vessels that allow nutrients to be absorbed into body tissues and the more capillaries we have the better the body becomes at utilising the nutrients for muscular repair. This expanded network of blood vessels also helps to clear waste products, particularly carbon dioxide from the food burning process. Efficient exchange of oxygen and nutrients in and carbon dioxide and waste out is paramount for fit and healthy body tissue.

In addition, the mitochondria (the energy factories) expand in size and number and require more energy. Once they have used up the glycogen (the stored glucose within the muscle cells and the liver), they call on the fat cells to release energy. Interval training provides significant benefits over *steady state* exercise and is more effective at burning fat because as with resistance training, the fat burning is prolonged after activity. This type of training involves intense effort for one minute followed by less intense effort for between one and four minutes. During the intense phase the lactic acid builds up quickly and during the less intense phase it is cleared from the blood and oxygen stores are replenished. This is repeated multiple times.

Here's an example: If you are a jogger, run as fast and as hard as you can for one minute then reduce your speed to a steady jog for between one and four minutes. Keep repeating until your 30 minutes is up. The same applies to rowing, cycling, swimming, skipping, using a mini trampoline or whatever gets your heart pumping. If you are on the treadmill in the gym, turn the knob to as fast as you can cope with for one minute then turn the speed down to a manageable jog for four minutes. A mere six repetitions and your 30 minutes of cardio are done. As you get fitter you can reduce the number of minutes between the intense phases to two minutes during the middle section of your workout.

Resistance training for 30 minutes on Monday, Wednesday and Friday (or Tuesday, Thursday and Saturday) and Interval Training for 30 minutes on the other three days with one day of rest suits many peoples' timetables, but you may prefer to do both in a one hour workout only three times a week (with one rest day between each). So which should you do first? Resistance followed by Interval appears to have the edge.

Since the body's preferred energy source is glucose that's what we should target first. Resistance Training does this. The body uses the glucose from recently consumed carbohydrates in the bloodstream followed by the stored glucose in the muscles and liver when we perform any type of anaerobic exercise. Resistance Training is anaerobic – it uses minimal oxygen and as fat can only be burned in the presence of oxygen the fat cells won't be mobilised into releasing their energy stores until after we stop. By the time we embark on the Interval Training, glycogen stores are pretty well used up and because Interval Training is aerobic (uses lots of oxygen) the body will have to call on the fat stores for energy. And, because of the intensity of both sessions the body will continue to burn calories for hours afterwards, requiring fat stores to continue providing some or much of that energy.

Unfit or Unused to Exercise? Don't worry, the principles of Resistance and Interval Training apply no matter where you start. Resistance Training is all about introducing some weights into your life and if you want to start with a couple of cans of baked beans you will still be creating *the force* and within a couple of weeks you can raise your game and seek out the litre bottles of water. From there it's all uphill. Similarly, Interval Training is all about moving as fast as you can manage for one minute followed by four minutes of slowing the pace. Walking is a great way to start – brisk for one minute, less intense for four. As you get fitter, your body will get acclimatised and you can push the intensity. Remember small changes make the difference.

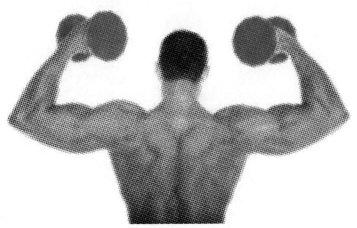

A Few Extra Fat Burning Strategies

The *successful 63%* who not only reached their fat loss goal but maintained it, shared a few of their secret strategies – some make biochemical sense, some are brilliant coping techniques and some are just plain wacky but they worked. It would be selfish of me not to share them. I have also added a few extras that may be helpful.

I always have 3 apples and a bag of almonds in my handbag. Apples (and pears) are high in pectin which helps reduce fat absorption and are also rich in soluble fibre which slows down the absorption of sugars into the bloodstream. Almonds are a great protein/essential fat combination. The two together make for a great fat burning, balanced and filling snack.

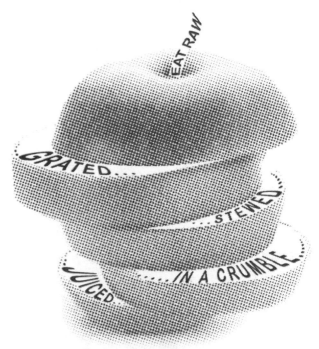

One day a week I only drink water and go to bed really early. As long as the day you pick is not full on, a day of *fasting* gives the digestive system a bit of a rest, allows the body to repair and can boost your metabolism for the next day or two. But, don't be tempted to *fast* for days on end without professional help. Your metabolic rate and consequently fat burning may slow down to compensate for the lack of food.

I can't give up cheese so I only eat it at the weekend. Full fat cheeses are high in calories and saturated fat and whilst they are a good source of calcium and add protein to the diet, they can pile on the pounds. Regarding them as a weekend treat means you don't deprive yourself of something you love but keeps you on track - good plan!

I use garlic, garlic paste and garlic oil a lot in my cooking. Garlic contains a substance called *allicin* which research has shown to have a significant protective quality to cells helping to reduce fatty deposits. Both garlic (and onions; also rich in allicin) have been linked to increasing our metabolic rate and insulin sensitivity. You may wish to experiment with garlic capsules to reduce the odour related to the regular ingestion of garlic however!

I love celery, particularly raw with nut butter or in soup. Celery is very low in calories and because it is also high in fibre, the digestive system burns more calories whilst digesting it; this is known as *diet induced thermogenesis* or DIT. Vegetables with less fibre and more water such as lettuce, peeled, canned vegetables and vegetable juices don't require the same amount of energy.

I snack on fish and vegetable sushi wrapped in seaweed. Seaweed is rich in iodine which feeds the thyroid gland, a major player in maintaining efficient metabolism. You might also wish to try kelp salt granules as an alternative to regular salt. They are rich in iodine, low in sodium and high in potassium, magnesium and other mineral salts which reduce the risk of high blood pressure.

I have a wheat-free week once a month. Wheat itself is not necessarily the devil; Western diets are overloaded with wheat products which can lead to intolerance. Bloating, flatulence and tiredness are some of the signs of a slight intolerance so a week a month of replacing wheat with oats and rye can certainly reduce the chances.

I have a teaspoon of apple cider vinegar before I eat. A couple of trials indicate that taking this vinegar before a meal creates a feeling of fullness so reducing the amount of food consumed. It can also aid digestion. But it is definitely an acquired taste!

I write down how I feel after I have eaten. This is a great tactic. Some foods make us feel lethargic and low, others give us energy, we feel *full of beans* and everything is achievable. Uncovering your list of positive foods allows you to get them into your day wherever possible whilst avoiding their negative counterparts which could be hindering fat loss.

I drink chilled green tea mixed with fresh fruit juice and sparkling water when hunger strikes. We often confuse hunger with thirst. A glass of water can seriously take the edge off our perceived hunger, but water can be unexciting. Caffeine-rich green tea mixed with deliciously sweet and vitamin-rich fresh fruit juice and topped up with fizzy water is a great idea. A filling, fat burning and altogether more exciting solution.

I double the size of my healthy snacks in the week before my period. Oestrogen levels are at their lowest and PMS is in full swing at this time of the month, triggering blood sugar fluctuations which make cravings hard to manage. Small and often is the way to go. Increasing the size of your healthy snacks may work for some, having more regular, but smaller healthy snacks may work for others - experiment and find what works for you.

Other slightly more unusual ploys adopted by my *successful 63%* include brushing your teeth or sucking an ice cube before you eat so you eat less, wearing blue tinted glasses as blue food is not as enticing as other colours and some even threw out all their 'fat' clothes, but that could prove pricey!

A few additional tactics to consider...

- When you keep it simple in the early stages you are more likely to stick to your plan.
- Every time you find yourself making excuses, note them down somewhere then try to avoid them.
- Going to bed an hour earlier and getting up an hour earlier means you are not tempted to eat late at night and you have time to exercise first thing in the morning.
- Goal setting is one of the greatest success strategies you can employ when it comes to fat loss. Write them down on post-it notes and stick them on the fridge or bathroom mirror, record them on your mobile phone etc and keep referring back to them.
- Eating on the run or in a rush creates stress within the body and turns on the fat storing mechanisms so take your time when you have the time.
- Having a protein shake can quickly satisfy hunger when your day is full on. Don't regard them as meal replacements however and check the label as many are loaded with sugar.
- Posting your diet on the internet and sharing your successes and concerns with others works for some. However, you may end up more confused than when you started!

- Spend time with slim people. Their shopping, cooking and eating habits can reveal a lot about how they stay that way.
- **Putting money in a jar/box every time you stick to your daily goal means you can afford to give yourself a reward from time to time – preferably not food!**
- When you go to the supermarket, park in the corner of the car park furthest away from the door so you have further to walk both ways (the heavier the shopping bags the more muscle you build!)
- **When parking in a multi-storey car park, go straight up to the top level and take the stairs both ways.**
- If you are a smoker and you go out of the office for a cigarette break, don't just stand outside and chat to other smokers – walk around the block.
- **Wearing a pedometer when out walking or jogging has been shown to result in people walking around a mile a day more than those who don't.**
- When you take the kids to the park, don't just stand and watch them, go on the swings with them or run around like they do.
- **When you have the dog on the lead, try and walk at the dog's pace rather than training it to walk at yours.**
- Don't take the lift unless you have loads to carry.
- **Even if you live or work on the top floor, take the stairs for at least two or three floors then the lift for the remainder (and NEVER take the lift down unless you are in a frantic rush).**
- Have more sex! Not only is it a great de-stressor but it burns up the calories (the more energetic, the more calories you burn; around 6-7kcals per minute is believed to be the average!)

There are a number of nutritional supplements that have been found, in conjunction with diet and lifestyle changes to encourage fat loss. Whilst they have shown encouraging results in a few studies, research is still in its infancy. In an effort to determine whether there may be one that can help burn fat more efficiently, the overriding recommendation is to consult a health professional. There are so many reasons why supplementation of any kind of fat loss accelerator may or may not work and self medication is not the way to go. It's all too easy to confuse our metabolism and not only will fat loss not result, but we could find ourselves a great deal lighter of pocket.

These Include:-

- **Conjugated Linoleic Acid (CLA)** – a growing body of research in the US and Europe shows that CLA reduces body fat and increases lean tissue.
- **Chromium** – preliminary research in animals and humans suggests that chromium picolinate increases fat loss by helping to maintain healthy blood sugar levels and curb cravings.
- **Hydroxycitric Acid (HCA)** – animal research indicates that HCA can suppress appetite and induce fat loss when taken before meals.
- **L-Carnitine** – preliminary studies suggest l-carnitine may be beneficial for fat loss when taken on a long term basis in combination with regular exercise.
- **Spirulina** – thought to nourish the thyroid gland which can be under-active in some overweight people.
- **5-HTP** – may play a role in raising serotonin levels which in turn reduces appetite.
- **7-Keto** – the association with fat loss is believed to be due to its ability to raise levels of T3, a thyroid hormone that plays a major role in metabolic rate.
- **Pyruvate** – has been noted to raise metabolic rate during the metabolism of protein and carbohydrates.
- **Fibre** – some studies show that supplementation with a source of fibre reduces appetite which in turn may influence satiety (the feeling of fullness) and fat loss.

Part 4. Fat Burning Action Plan

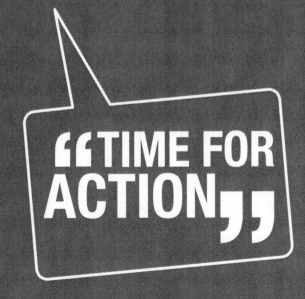

Get hooked on soup for fat loss. It's fast, filling, nourishing, delicious, easy-on-the-pocket and fat burning. It truly ticks all the boxes.

2 Weeks in the *Fast Lane*

Repetition may work for exercise and learning French verbs but not for successful fat loss. My research clearly indicates that when a diet is too repetitive, boredom quickly manifests itself, we feel deprived, we start to obsess about food and cravings invade our day. This diet offers plenty of variety so I urge you to experiment with the choices offered and find the ones that fit your individual tastes and priorities to ensure that boredom doesn't become an issue - flexibility pays dividends. The following points are important and are an integral part of this energising, mood-boosting, fast fat burning plan:-

- You have to make it a priority
- You have to eat something every 2-3 hours
- You have to start it on any day of the week other than a Monday
- You have to bin the *white stuff* and only include starchy carbohydrates before 6pm
- You have to get half an hour's physical activity into your day
- You have to drink water every 2-3 hours
- You have to keep it simple

Why should you make it a priority? Convincing your body to use fat stores for energy in super-quick time requires careful manipulation of the types of foods you eat so you have to treat it as a project and focus.

Why should you eat something every 2-3 hours? To keep the fat burning furnace firing all day, every day and to ensure you body swerve the energy dips and cravings. When you are tired and hungry resolve takes a dive.

Why should you start on any day other than Monday? The *successful 63%* largely agreed that when you start a diet on a Monday you see the weekend as an opportunity to pig out before the deprivation starts – hardly a recipe for success. Also, you may have noticed that Monday is the only day of the week that seems to attract negative adjectives like blue, gloomy and depressing. Why risk it? Do your planning and shopping at the beginning of the week and start midweek.

Why should you bin the white foods? They are an instant but short-lived energy source, provide few nutrients and don't fill you up for long. They raise the level of glucose in the bloodstream too quickly and in an effort to regain the necessary balance the sugars are shipped off for immediate use or stored in the liver, muscles and fat cells until required. If you want the fat cells to shrink you can't afford to give them the opportunity to expand their storage facilities. They have to be badgered into releasing their stores to provide energy. Keeping the sugar level balanced by eating colourful nutrient-rich foods can help to achieve this; white foods make it a whole lot harder.

Why should you avoid starchy carbohydrates after 6pm? Because they provide energy during the day when you are active but can leave you feeling bloated and uncomfortable at bedtime. They may also promote fat storage through the night (the jury is still out on this one at time of publication but why risk it?).

Why should you get half an hour's physical activity into your day? Because working muscles need lots of energy (20-50 times more than they do at rest) so the fat stores are forced into action yet again. And if you *get physical* first thing in the morning you fat burn more efficiently for as much as 8 hours afterwards (some suggest it may be as much as 24 hours).

Why should you drink water every 2-3 hours? Because every chemical reaction that takes place in the body 24/7 from extracting nutrients from food to encouraging fat burning needs water to get a result.

Why should you keep it simple? Contrary to the spin surrounding some diets, losing fat is not easy, effortless or care-free. You have to commit. Whilst the debate rages on, many successful dieters agree that too much choice can be a major stumbling block in the early stages. This plan combines maximum nourishment with minimum choice to ensure compliance and success rather than confusion and frustration. Studies show that while extensive choices are initially appealing, subsequent satisfaction and motivation are more often achieved when choice is reduced but variety predominates.

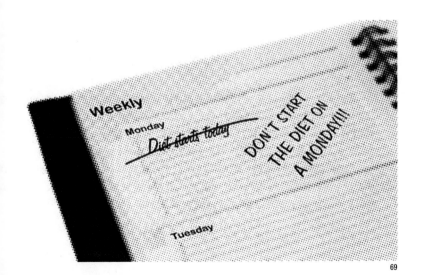

So what do you have to do?

1. Get up half an hour earlier, have a small, rich coffee and get physical for 30 minutes
2. Skin brush before your shower and eat fruit and drink only juiced fruit/smoothies and still or sparkling water until late morning
3. If you need a hot drink have fresh black coffee, black, green, red bush or herb/fruit tea before or after your late morning snack without milk or sugar
4. Have a late morning snack
5. Have soup and salad around lunchtime
6. If you need another hot drink follow the recommendations above (not fruit tea)
7. Have a mid afternoon snack
8. Have a light meal around dinner time with no starchy carbohydrates
9. Have a small bedtime snack at least 30 mins before you go to bed (only if you are really hungry or you find you are waking up in the wee small hours and can't get back to sleep)

1. Get Physical

Muscle is what is known as active tissue so it really munches its way through the calories. Fat cells, on the other hand are more than happy to store energy until they are called into action. So if you want to wake up those fat cells, you have to maintain, or even better gain muscle mass. Half an hour a day, six days a week – can't be that hard (and don't forget your shot of coffee if you exercise first thing).

2. Skin Brush

Lightly brushing the skin with a dry brush or loofah stimulates the circulation, removes dead skin cells and promotes elimination. Start brushing at your feet and brush towards the heart, then brush from the fingertips up to the shoulders and toward the heart (don't forget the soles of your feet and the palms of your hands). Use small strokes and a gentle pressure - you're not brushing the dog. Avoid the face and neck area and any damaged or bruised skin. Jump into the shower and have a good rinse to get rid of the dead skin cells before soaping. If you are brave enough you can turn the shower to cold (but not freezing) for a few minutes before you dry off to encourage your body to launch into a bit more fat burning to keep warm. If you have an ongoing health condition or are on medication, check with your doctor before considering this rude awakening!

3. Get Fruity

There are a host of reasons why permanent weight loss is such a struggle but a sluggish or inefficient digestive system is one of the most common obstacles. Fruits provide a quick energy source and are bursting with nourishment but when consumed with other foods they can cause havoc for some. By being trapped in the stomach for too long they undergo fermentation which can not only upset the digestive process of other foods but also reduce the nutritional value of the fruit. When you eat them on their own and on an empty stomach they take a mere 30 minutes to pass through the stomach and while reaping all their cleansing and nourishing benefits you avoid possible bloating, flatulence or intestinal irritation that you may be all too familiar with.

After your 30 minutes of exercise and every hour thereafter through to late morning (11.30/noon) have fresh fruit, juiced fruits and fresh fruit smoothies. Select from any of the following, make sure you don't add any proteins or fats (watch out for yoghurt in shop-bought smoothies), go for plenty of variety and wait until late morning before you have your regular cup of tea/coffee.

Fresh fruits straight from the tree/bush
Keep the peel on where possible and give them a good scrub before eating whole or chopping, slicing or dicing. Aim for as much colour as possible throughout the morning and be generous with your portions.

Fresh fruit juices
Citrus fruits are born to be juiced. Half a few oranges and get as much as you can out of them (an electric or battery operated citrus press is a cheap and highly effective bonus here). Add lemon, lime, mandarin, tangerine, Clementine and grapefruit to the mix to ring the changes.

Smoothies
All you need is a blender and you're good to go. Sling a few ice cubes and a teacup of water into the blender then add fruits of choice. Berries, cherries (if you can be bothered to stone them), melon, peaches and nectarines, kiwi, tropical fruits like mango, papaya, pineapple, passion fruit and pawpaw, bananas, apples, pears, apricots, plums, grapes, figs, tomatoes (yes, they are a fruit) and of course citrus fruits all blend well. See *Quick Fix Fruits* in the recipe section for delicious combinations. Bags of frozen fruits are great for smoothies if you don't have time to chop, peel and slice. Strain the juice through a sieve before drinking if you don't like the seedy/gritty bits and add more water if it's too thick and gloopy. Don't down them in one go, sip them slowly and savour the flavours.

Juices
If you already own a juicer, get it out of the cupboard and go for it. You lose a whole lot less of the goodness of the fruits (vitamins, minerals and fibre) when you juice them. Sip them slowly while you are cleaning the machine or pop the juice in a thermos and sip throughout the morning. If you don't have a juicer, see if you can find a juice bar near your work or home and test a few of their fruit combinations but remember; only fruits, no added extras.

Bottled juices and smoothies
These provide the least amount of goodness as they have been processed to allow them a few days shelf life, but there are plenty out there that have been sympathetically produced to provide you with as fresh a juice as possible. Generally speaking, price is a good guide - the more expensive they are, the more goodness has been retained and because they are less processed they don't have a long shelf life. You will often find them discounted because their 'use by' date is perilously close – grab them.

4. Have a Hot Drink if You Need it

If you usually have coffee or tea in the morning, you may be struggling by late morning. Now is the time to have your cuppa. Choose good quality black coffee from ground beans, black, green, red bush or herb/fruit tea before or after your late morning snack and don't add milk or sugar.

Have a soya milk latte with no sugar occasionally if the need for a milky drink is intense.

5. Have a Late Morning Snack

Choose one of the following and stick to the *Suggested 7 Day Plan* or select from the *Quick Fix Snacks* on page 102:-

- Small pack of unsalted nuts (no dried fruit)
- Cold, cooked chicken leg or breast (skin removed), a couple of tomatoes and a small handful of fresh nuts
- Couple of oatcakes spread with tinned, mashed salmon topped with cucumber slices
- A tray or pack of raw baby vegetables with a small pot of hummus
- A tray or pack of raw baby vegetables with a small pot of guacamole
- Bowl of mixed olives with feta cheese cubes or olives stuffed with anchovies or almonds
- 3 bean salad from the 'deli' section of most supermarkets (or make your own)

6. Get Soupy (and have a small salad)

It's filling, it's fast, it's nutritious and it's widely available. Have a bowl or mug of soup around lunchtime every day. You can also have soup as your late morning or mid afternoon snack or in the evening if time is the enemy or you are going out. If you do opt for soup for your evening meal occasionally or within 4 hours of going to bed, ensure that it is a vegetable, meat, poultry or fish combination with no starchy carbohydrates included (rice, barley, beans, lentils, noodles etc.) Also, experiment with chilled soups if we are having a rare, but welcome heat wave.

Home made soups

If you can find the time, these are the healthiest option as you know exactly what's going into them and you can put as few or as many ingredients in as you wish. Experiment with the soups in the recipe section (and remember to leave out the starchy carbohydrates if you are having a bowl after 6pm).

Ready made soups

There are so many varieties available that you could have three different soups a day, seven days a week for at least a month and never have the same one twice. However, there are a great many that are high in fat, salt or sugar (or all three), so label reading is vital. Head for the vegetabley, meaty, fishy, beany ones and body swerve the creamy ones (and as before avoid the ones with starchy carbohydrates after 6pm). Be particularly vigilant about packet and tinned soups and follow the food label guidelines on the next page.

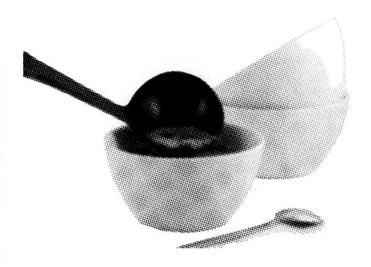

Look at the *per 100g* column rather than the *per serving* column and follow the guidelines:-

Spot the Sugar – where it says Carbohydrates: *of which sugars*, 10g is high, 2g is low. Aim for a maximum of 4g.

Spot the Saturated Fat – where is says Fats: *of which saturates*, 5g is high, 1g is low. Aim for a maximum of 2g.

Spot the Salt – where it says Salt or *salt equivalent*, 1.5g is high, 0.3g is low. Aim for a maximum of 0.6g.

Spot the Sodium – where it says Sodium, 0.5g is high, 0.1g is low. Aim for a maximum of 0.2g.

Super quick soup
A spoonful of miso paste or a sachet of miso soup dissolved in boiling water is not only warming and tasty but very nutritious and can keep hunger pangs at bay. Same goes for a mug of *Marigold Swiss Vegetable Bouillon*. Keep a tub handy and opt for the low salt version. You can also combine the two. There are scores of quick soups and cuppa soups on the supermarket shelves but many of them are scarily salt-ridden. Again, check the label. However, if you are following the recommended eating plan and adding herbs and spices to your food for added flavour instead of salt, your salt intake should reduce drastically so your soup choice needn't be the enemy. Just keep an eye on it and follow the salt and sodium guidelines above.

Have a Small Salad
There are lots of salad suggestions in the recipe section (and dressings). If you opt for bought/ready made salads, bin the little pack of salad dressing and replace with a mix of olive nut or seed oil and a squirt of lemon/lime juice.

7. Have a Hot Drink if You Need it

Follow the mid morning recommendations before or after your mid afternoon snack but avoid fruit teas.

8. Have a Mid Afternoon Snack

Choose one of the following and stick to the *Suggested 7 Day Plan* or select from the *Quick Fix Snacks* on page 102:-

- Small pack of mixed, unsalted nuts and seeds (no dried fruit)
- Couple of brown Ryvita with chopped boiled egg mixed with natural live yoghurt and chopped herbs
- A tray or pack of raw baby vegetables with a small pot of natural cottage cheese
- A tray or pack or raw baby vegetables with a small pot of salsa
- A cold boiled egg and a couple of slices of cooked ham
- A couple of sticks of celery filled with nut butter (almond, cashew, hazelnut, walnut, macadamia or peanut)
- A grain bar – the *Food Doctor* and *Gillian McKeith's* are good choices (go for the ones without dried fruit)

NB – buy omega 3-rich eggs whenever possible. The hens that lay these eggs are fed on a diet rich in seeds that provide the essential omega 3 fats that help to promote fat burning - and they taste great.

9. Have a Light Meal Around Dinner Time

This is the time of the day to say no to starchy carbohydrates. The combination of a decent portion of good quality protein, some essential fats and plenty of vegetables provide a filling meal that gives your body everything it needs to rest, repair and fat burn all night.

You will find light meal suggestions in the *7 day plan* and also in the recipe section.

If you are only able to fit your half hour of exercise into the early evening and usually have your meal afterwards, you can add a cupful of brown rice, barley, couscous, beans or lentils, a baked sweet potato or sweet potato chips (scrub, don't peel and cut into generous chips, paint with olive oil and bake in a moderate oven until crispy round the edges and succulent within).

Have at least 3 different steamed, grilled, stir fried or roasted vegetables (not starchy potatoes, root vegetables or corn) and/or a large mixed salad. Top your vegetables or salad with roasted mixed nuts or seeds or mixed bean sprouts and drizzle with nut or seed oil (avocado, sesame, sunflower, pumpkin, walnut, flax, hemp etc.) and a squeeze of lemon/ lime juice. See *Quick Fix Salads* and *Quick Fix Vegetables* in the recipe section.

10. Have a Bedtime Snack

Only if you are really hungry or you find you can't get to sleep or you regularly wake up in the wee small hours and can't get back to sleep. The following food combinations are rich in the amino acid, tryptophan which encourages the production of the *sleepy* chemical, serotonin plus if your blood sugar is all over the place can help to get the balance right overnight. Have your snack at least 30 minutes before you go to bed. You will probably find after a few days in the *fast lane* you will be sleeping better and it won't be required:-

- A couple of mini oatcakes with nut or seed butter and a couple of slices of cold turkey breast
- A mug of *Green & Black's* hot chocolate made with soya milk
- A small tub of natural cottage cheese with a handful of mixed seeds
- One egg lightly scrambled on an oatcake
- A small carton of natural live yoghurt with a swirl of honey
- 2 or 3 squares of dark chocolate (70% cocoa solids minimum) and a few shavings of parmesan cheese
- A small plate of porridge made with water and topped with a spoonful of Manuka honey

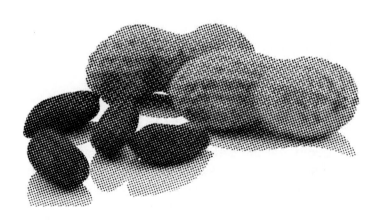

Suggested 7 Day Plan

IMPORTANT: Whilst soups, juices and smoothies feature daily in this plan, **it is not a liquid diet**. You may wish to substitute soup for your late morning or mid afternoon snack occasionally and even for your evening meal if time is short or you are going out, but **don't fall into the trap of living on fruit juice and soup day after day**.

Stick to the plan below as closely as possible for 2 weeks but don't panic if time is against you and you haven't planned ahead. The *Quick Fix Rescue Plan* at the back of the book provides shop bought and on-the-go strategies that won't wreck your diet. Photocopy it or download it from my website and keep it near at hand to get you out of trouble.

After 2 weeks you can continue the plan for as long as you wish if you are the type who likes to stick fairly rigidly to a plan **OR** you can play around with the recipe/snack suggestions (and the *Quick Fix Rescue Plan* strategies) to suit your tastes, your timetable and your commitments. Just make sure you keep it varied. As mentioned previously, repetition can lead to boredom and boredom can lead to a loss of resolve - don't risk it!

And remember:-

- **eat only fruit** until 11.30am/noon.
- have a bowl of soup at lunchtime.
- **have a creative mix of salad stuffs** with your soup (see salad suggestions page 100-101)
- **avoid starchy carbohydrates after 6pm** (no rice, pasta, bread, potatoes, sweet potatoes, beans, lentils, root vegetables or corn). See carbohydrate choices on page 85 if you exercise in the evening.
- **have at least 3 vegetables or a big salad** with your evening meal (see salad suggestions on page 100-101

and vegetable suggestions on page 111)

- **have a bedtime snack** only if you are really hungry or sleep is a struggle.
- **swap mid morning and mid afternoon snacks** around freely or just concentrate on the ones you like best (see *Quick Fix Snacks* on page 102 for full list).
- **get back on track** as quickly as you can if things go awry - it was merely a blip!

First thing in the morning

- Double espresso (no milk or sugar)
- 30 minutes exercise followed by a large glass of water
- Skin brush and shower

Every hour until late morning (11.30am/noon)

- Fresh fruits, juiced fruits, fruit smoothies and fresh fruit juices

Late morning and mid afternoon

- Hot drink

Throughout the day (every couple of hours)

- Still or sparkling water

Day 1

Morning	Fresh fruits, juiced fruits, fruit smoothies and fresh fruit juices
Late Morning	Small pack of unsalted nuts
Lunchtime	Beef Broth with Pearl Barley (p90) or Lamb and Bean Soup (p94) Salad (p100)
Mid Afternoon	Ryvita and chopped egg
Evening	Fish Fillets Thai-Style (p104) or Very Quick Salmon (p109) Vegetables/Salad (p111 and 101) (+ starchy carbohydrate if you exercise in the evening*)
Bedtime	Oatcakes and turkey slices (p79)

Day 2

Morning	Fresh fruits, juiced fruits, fruit smoothies and fresh fruit juices
Late Morning	Oatcakes with tinned salmon and cucumber
Lunchtime	Pea, Mint and Lettuce Soup (p91) or Spicy Red Pepper and Sweet Potato Soup (p91) Salad (p100)
Mid Afternoon	Grain Bar
Evening	Frittata (p108) or Very Quick Omelette (p110) Vegetables/Salad (p111 and 101) (+ starchy carbohydrate if you exercise in the evening*)
Bedtime	Hot chocolate (p79)

Day 3

Morning	Fresh fruits, juiced fruits, fruit smoothies and fresh fruit juices
Late Morning	Raw baby vegetables with hummus
Lunchtime	Chinese Little Gem and Chicken/Tofu Soup (p93) or Chicken and Vegetable Soup (p98) Salad (p100)
Mid Afternoon	Cold boiled egg and ham

Evening	Tomato, Squash and Spinach Curry (p104) or
	Very Quick Tofu (p110) or
	Very Quick Mackerel (p110)
	Vegetables/Salad (p111 and 101)
	(+ starchy carbohydrate if you exercise in the evening*)
Bedtime	Porridge and honey (p79)

Day 4

Morning	Fresh fruits, juiced fruits, fruit smoothies and fresh fruit juices
Late Morning	Cold cooked chicken, tomatoes and fresh nuts
Lunchtime	Lamb and Bean Soup (p94) or
	Beef Broth with Pearl Barley (p90)
	Salad (p100)
Mid Afternoon	Raw baby vegetables with salsa
Evening	Spicy Prawns (p106) or
	Very Quick Prawns (p110)
	Vegetables/Salad (p111 and 101)
	(+ starchy carbohydrate if you exercise in the evening*)
Bedtime	Chocolate and cheese (p79)

Day 5

Morning	Fresh fruits, juiced fruits, fruit smoothies and fresh fruit juices
Late Morning	3 Bean Salad
Lunchtime	Long-Stemmed Broccoli Soup (p92) or
	Spinach and Watercress Soup (p95)
	Salad (p100)
Mid Afternoon	Raw baby vegetables with cottage cheese
Evening	Beef/Lamb Stew (p105) or
	Very Quick Lamb (p109)
	Vegetables/Salad (p111 and 101)
	(+ starchy carbohydrate if you exercise in the evening*)
Bedtime	Yoghurt and honey (p79)

Day 6

Morning   Fresh fruits, juiced fruits, fruit smoothies and
              fresh fruit juices
Late Morning   Mixed olives with feta cheese or stuffed olives
Lunchtime   Spicy Pepper and Sweet Potato Soup (p91)
              or Lentil Soup/Spicy Lentil Soup (p96)
              Salad (p100)
Mid Afternoon Small pack of fresh nuts and seeds
Evening   Beef Stroganoff (p107) or
              Very Quick Pork (p109) or
              Very Quick Chicken (p109)
              Vegetables/Salad (p111 and 101)
              (+ starchy carbohydrate if you exercise in the evening*)
Bedtime   Cottage cheese and seeds (p79)

Day 7

Morning   Fresh fruits, juiced fruits, fruit smoothies and
              fresh fruit juices
Late Morning   Raw baby vegetables with guacamole
Lunchtime   Tasty Fish Soup (p97) or
              Chicken and Vegetable Soup (p98)
              Salad (p100)
Mid Afternoon Celery sticks with nut butter
Evening   Turkey Burgers (p106) or
              Very Quick Burgers (p110)
              Vegetables/Salad (p111 and 101)
              (+ starchy carbohydrate if you exercise in the evening*)
Bedtime   Oatcake and scrambled egg (p79)

*Starchy carbohydrate choices to include if you exercise in the evening (or have an action-packed night ahead!)

- cup of quick-cook couscous
- cup of quick-cook brown rice
- cup of quick-cook quinoa
- cup of tinned, cooked beans (kidney, haricot, barlotti, black-eyed, cannellini, flageolet, broad beans, chickpeas or mixed)
- cup of tinned, cooked lentils (red, green, Puy or mixed)
- small baked sweet potato
- baked sweet potato chips (cut a small sweet potato into fat chips, coat with olive oil, put on a roasting tray in a hot oven and bake until cooked through and crispy outside)

If you don't have the time (or the inclination) to cook fresh, shop-bought soups, juices, smoothies and salads are fine as long as you follow the guidelines on pages 71-76. And, always keep the Quick Fix Rescue Plan near at hand when you are out and about - particularly in the evening.

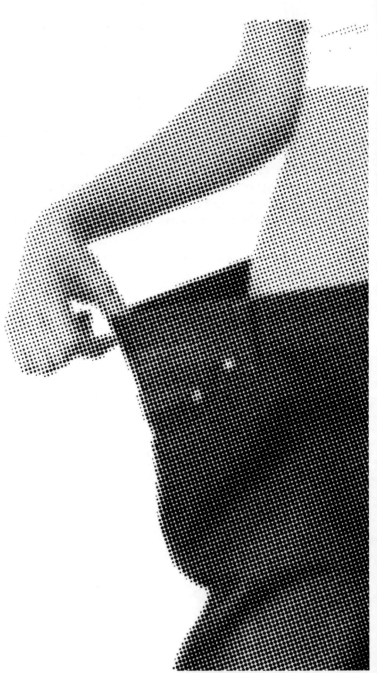

Part 5. Fat Burning Recipes

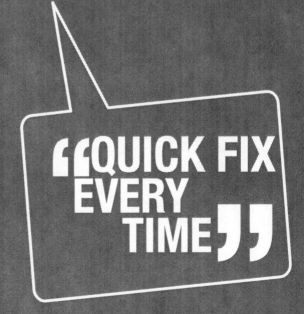

"QUICK FIX EVERY TIME"

Make a little more than you need today and you are ahead of the game tomorrow. Sounds easy - it is.

Quick Fix Fruits

Juices + Smoothies

Less is definitely more when it comes to fruit drinks. It is tempting to throw in every tired-looking specimen that is lurking in the fruit bowl and the desire to sling in half a banana to give it a bit more substance can be fierce but can kill many a good smoothie. A deliciously, satisfying fruit drink relies on just a few ingredients but combination is key.

Get the blender out, sling in a few ice cubes and a teacup of cold water then add your fruits of choice, chopped into bite-sized pieces (remember to keep the skin on and just give them a good scrub, wherever possible). Whizz slowly at first until the ingredients start to come together then go for maximum power until smooth. Add the extras (fruit juice/ herbs/spices/flavourings) then blitz again briefly. Add cold water if you need to thin it down, strain the juice through a sieve if you don't like the seedy/gritty bits and sip slowly whilst you rinse out the blender. Put any extra in a flask for later in the morning.

Here are a few winning combinations that take a maximum of 15 minutes.

Apple and Blueberry with Fresh Lemon Juice and Cinnamon
Apple, Raspberry and Grapes with Fresh Orange Juice
Apple and Plum with Morello Cherry Juice and a drizzle of Honey
Grapefruit, Passion Fruit and Pineapple
Tangerine, Strawberry and Banana
Mango and Mixed Berries with Fresh Lime Juice
Watermelon and Cantaloupe Melon with cold Green Tea
Rhubarb, Orange, Fresh Ginger and Mint leaves
Peach, Raspberry and Redcurrants with Rose Water
Pear, Melon and Blackberries with Ground Black Pepper
Tomato, Orange and Apple with Fresh Basil

These combinations feature fresh fruits but the whole exercise can become even swifter if you have a few bags of frozen fruits in the freezer; Tropical Fruit Mixes, Summer Berry Mixes, Rhubarb, Cranberries, Blueberries, Blackberries, Blackcurrants, Redcurrants, Pineapples, Apples. You can use them straight from the freezer which means you can dispense with the ice cubes.

Other fresh juices, herbs, spices and flavourings you might like to add to your fruit selection include apple, pineapple, passionfruit, cranberry or grapefruit juice, fresh marjoram, lemon thyme or spearmint, grated nutmeg or powdered allspice, vanilla essence, balsamic or fruit vinegars and don't forget fruit flavoured vodkas for those rare occasions when your day is not overloaded with work or domestic commitments!

Quick Fix Soups

Beef Broth with Pearl Barley
50 mins/serves 2

Ingredients

1 tbsp olive oil
250g lean stewing steak, cut into small cubes
2 tsp balsamic vinegar
2 tsp Worcestershire sauce
1 small onion, finely chopped
1 carrot, finely diced
1 stalk celery, finely sliced
2 tsp *Marigold Vegetable Bouillon* powder in 500ml hot water
75g pearl barley
1 small bay leaf
1 small sprig fresh rosemary
Handful chopped fresh parsley
Sea salt and freshly ground black pepper

Method

1. Warm the oil in a medium-sized pan and gently brown the meat over a medium heat.

2. Add the balsamic vinegar and Worcestershire sauce, turn up the heat and stir vigorously until most of the liquid has gone.
3. Add the vegetables, bay leaf and rosemary, put the lid on and cook over a low heat until vegetables are tender, about 20 mins.
4. Add the stock and bring to the boil.
5. Add the pearl barley and parsley and simmer until the barley is tender (25 mins).
6. Take the pan off the heat and remove the bay leaf and rosemary. Season to taste.
7. Whizz with a hand blender to preferred texture. Add boiling water to thin if necessary.

Pea, Mint and Lettuce Soup
20 mins/serves 2

Ingredients

2 tsp *Marigold Vegetable Bouillon* powder in 500ml hot water
250g frozen peas
6 large green lettuce leaves, washed and shredded
Handful fresh mint leaves
Sea salt and freshly ground black pepper

Method

1. Put the stock in a good sized pan and bring to the boil. Add the peas and simmer until tender (10 mins).
2. Add mint leaves and shredded lettuce and simmer for a couple more minutes.
3. Whizz with a hand blender until smooth and season to taste.

Spicy Pepper and Sweet Potato Soup
40 mins/serves 2

Ingredients

1 tbsp olive oil

1 small onion, finely sliced and 1 small garlic clove, crushed
1 stalk celery, finely sliced
1 small red pepper (or ½ large), de-seeded and finely sliced
1 small yellow pepper (or ½ large), de-seeded and finely sliced
1 small orange pepper (or ½ large), de-seeded and finely sliced
1 small sweet potato (or ½ large), peeled and finely diced
1 small tin (or ½ large), chopped tomatoes
½ fresh chilli or 1 tsp powdered chilli
2 tsp *Marigold Vegetable Bouillon* powder in 500ml hot water
Sea salt and freshly ground black pepper

Method

1. Warm the olive oil in a medium-sized pan, add all the vegetables and fresh chilli if using and cook over a medium heat until tender.
2. Add the tomatoes, chilli powder (if not using fresh) and vegetable stock.
3. Bring to the boil and simmer for a further 5 mins then mash well to give a chunky texture or blend if you prefer a smooth soup. Season to taste.

Long-Stemmed Broccoli Soup
30 mins/serves 2

Ingredients

200g long-stemmed broccoli, trimmed and roughly sliced
50g sun-dried tomatoes in oil, roughly chopped (keep oil)
1 small onion, finely sliced
1 clove garlic, finely sliced
Small pinch chilli powder
2 tsp *Marigold Vegetable Bouillon* powder in 500ml hot water
Small bunch fresh parsley, finely chopped
Sea salt and freshly ground black pepper

Method

1. Heat the oil from the sun-dried tomatoes and gently sauté the onion until soft.

2. Add the sun-dried tomatoes, garlic and chilli powder half way through and stir frequently. Add the broccoli and continue to toss for a few minutes.
3. Add most of the stock and gently simmer for 10 mins or until the broccoli is tender.
4. Use a hand blender or whizz in a food processor until you have a nice chunky consistency, using the remaining stock or a little boiling water if the soup is too thick.
5. Stir through the parsley, season to taste and add a splash of lemon juice.

Chinese Little Gem and Chicken/Tofu Soup

35 mins/serves 2

Ingredients

1 tbsp olive oil
1 small clove garlic, crushed
2cm piece fresh ginger, peeled and finely sliced
6 spring onions, white part chopped finely, green part cut into 5cm pieces
2 tsp *Marigold Vegetable Bouillon* powder in 500ml hot water
2 small chicken breasts finely sliced along the grain and/or 50g tofu, cubed
1 little gem lettuce, finely sliced
Good splash Tamari or light Soy Sauce

Method

1. Warm the oil, add the garlic, ginger and white spring onion and sauté for 2 mins.
2. Add the stock and bring to a simmer, add the chicken and/or tofu, green part of the spring onion, lettuce, Tamari/Soy Sauce and cook gently for 5 mins.

Bok choy is a good substitute for the lettuce and if you want to bulk the soup out a bit add a tablespoon of brown rice and cook well in the stock before adding the chicken/tofu.

Lamb and Bean Soup
40 mins/serves 2

Ingredients

100g lean lamb mince
½ tbsp Worcestershire sauce
½ tsp each of ground cumin, paprika and chilli
1 tbsp olive oil
1 small onion, finely chopped
1 clove garlic, finely chopped
1 small red pepper, thinly sliced
1 carrot sliced into thin strips
½ tin black-eyed or canellini beans, drain but keep the liquid
1 baby cabbage or 1 little gem lettuce, finely sliced
2 tomatoes skinned or 2 tinned plum tomatoes, chopped
2 tsp *Marigold Vegetable Bouillon* powder in 500ml hot water
Fresh parsley or coriander leaves
Sea salt and freshly ground black pepper

Method

1. Brown the meat in a non-stick pan, add the Worcestershire sauce and keep stirring until the meat is browned and the liquid is absorbed. Add spices and stir well.
2. Heat the oil in another pan, add the onion and garlic and cook until softened, add the pepper and carrot and cook for a further 5 mins.
3. Whizz one third of the beans in a food processor.
4. Add the bean liquid, most of the stock, puréed beans and cabbage (if using) and simmer gently for 15 mins.
5. Add the tomatoes, remaining beans and lettuce (if not using cabbage) and cook for a further 5 mins.
6. Add more stock if the soup is too thick.
7. Season to taste and garnish with finely chopped parsley or coriander.

Spinach and Watercress Soup
20 mins/serves 2

Ingredients

1 tbsp olive oil
1 small onion, roughly chopped
2 tsp *Marigold Vegetable Bouillon* powder in 500ml hot water
1 level dessertspoon porridge oats
½ bag fresh spinach
½ bag fresh watercress
Sea salt and freshly ground black pepper
Lemon juice

Method

1. Warm the oil and sauté the onion until soft.
2. Add the stock and porridge, bring to the boil then simmer until porridge is cooked (10-15 mins).
3. Add spinach and watercress, bring soup back to the boil then use hand blender until you have a smooth consistency.
4. Season and add lemon juice to taste.

Lentil Soup
35mins/serves 2

Ingredients

1 thin leek, well washed and finely sliced
1 stick celery, finely sliced
2 large carrots, scrubbed and diced
2 tsp *Marigold Vegetable Bouillon* powder in 500ml hot water
75g red split lentils, rinsed
Small bunch curly parsley, finely chopped
Sea salt and freshly ground black pepper

Method

1. Put leek, celery and carrot into a good sized pan, add

stock and bring to boil. Turn the heat down and add the lentils.
2. Simmer for 20 mins or until vegetables are tender and the lentils are cooked through.
3. Add the parsley, then mash to a nice chunky texture or whizz with a hand blender until smooth.
4. Season to taste.

Spicy Red Lentil Soup
40 mins/serves 2

Ingredients

1 tsp olive oil
1 tsp paprika
1 tsp turmeric
Small pinch cinnamon
Small pinch cayenne pepper
1 small onion, finely chopped
1 medium carrot, scrubbed and diced
1 small red pepper, de-seeded and sliced
75g red split lentils, rinsed
½ tin chopped tomatoes
2 tsp *Marigold Vegetable Bouillon* powder in 500ml hot water
1 tsp dried basil or Italian Mixed Herbs
1 small bay leaf
Sea salt and freshly ground black pepper

Method

1. Warm the oil and lightly sauté spices.
2. Add vegetables and lentils and stir to coat with spices.
3. Add tomatoes, stock, basil and bay leaf.
4. Bring to the boil and simmer for 40 mins or until lentils and vegetables are cooked.
5. Remove the bay leaf, season to taste and add more water if necessary.

Tasty Fish Soup

20 mins/serves 2

Ingredients

1 tbsp light olive oil
1 clove garlic, finely sliced
½ tsp peeled, grated fresh ginger
¼ tsp red chilli, seeds removed, very finely chopped
1 tsp bashed, finely chopped lemongrass (or use ready chopped from a jar)
200g fresh crab meat (tinned if you are in a rush)
500ml fish stock (most supermarkets have handy tubs)
150ml coconut milk
1 tbsp Thai fish sauce, or to taste
50g uncooked shelled de-veined prawns
1 spring onion, finely sliced
Lemon juice
1 tbsp chopped fresh coriander
Freshly ground black pepper

Method

1. Heat the oil in a large saucepan over a medium heat then add the garlic, ginger, chilli, lemongrass and crab meat and sauté for 4-5 mins.
2. Pour in the stock, coconut milk and fish sauce, increase the heat to high and bring to the boil.
3. Reduce the heat to low, tip in the prawns and simmer gently for 1-2 mins, until the prawns are pink and cooked through.
4. Stir in the spring onion, lemon juice and coriander and season to taste.

Chicken and Vegetable Soup
40 mins/serves 2

Ingredients

2 tsp *Marigold Vegetable Bouillon* powder in 500ml hot water
2 small skinless chicken breasts
1 tbsp olive oil
1 small onion, finely chopped
1 garlic clove, finely chopped
2 small carrots, finely diced
1 celery stick, finely sliced
2 tbsp finely chopped fresh parsley
Sea salt and freshly ground black pepper

Method

1. Bring stock to a simmer in a medium-sized pan.
2. Add chicken and simmer very gently, uncovered for 6 mins.
3. Remove pan from heat, cover and let stand until chicken is cooked through, about 15 mins.
4. Transfer chicken to a plate to cool. Reserve poaching liquid.
5. While chicken is poaching, sauté onion in oil in another pan over a moderate heat until softened but not brown.
6. Add garlic and sauté for a further minute.
7. Add carrots and celery and sauté, covered, stirring occasionally, until soft, 8 to 10 mins.
8. Add poaching liquid and simmer, covered until vegetables are tender then remove from heat.
9. While vegetables are cooking, shred chicken and stir into soup just before serving with the parsley.
10. Season to taste.

Toppings for Soups

- A spoonful of pesto.
- A spoonful of live natural yoghurt or tzatziki.
- A dollop of hummus.
- A spoonful of salsa.
- A spoonful of whole grain mustard.
- A swirl of nut or seed oil.
- A swirl of seasoned olive oil (chilli, basil etc).
- A drizzle of truffle oil.
- A dash of Worcestershire sauce, soy sauce or balsamic vinegar.
- A handful of bean sprouts.
- A handful of toasted nuts and/or seeds.
- Chopped fresh herbs.
- Dried, powdered or flaked spices.
- Grated fresh coconut.
- Grated fresh ginger.
- A spoonful of coconut cream.
- Very finely diced fresh red or green chilli (de-seeded).
- Finely chopped fresh or sun-dried tomatoes.
- Finely diced fresh apple.
- Caramelised very thinly sliced onion rings or leek circles.
- Crispy, lean bacon or pancetta bits.
- Crispy seaweed or nori flakes.
- Lightly-steamed asparagus tips.
- Chopped chives or spring onions.
- Grated Swiss cheese.

Quick Fix Salads at Lunchtime
(starchy carbohydrates **may** be included)

If you have time to make your own:-

Base – all kinds of lettuce, spinach leaves, watercress, rocket fresh parsley and mixed herbs, sliced fennel, spring onions, sliced red onions, Chinese leaves, bok choy, mustard cress, baby gem lettuce, chicory leaves, celery leaves, chives, shredded cabbage celery, finely sliced leeks.

Next – tomatoes (fresh and sun-dried), cucumber, bean sprouts green beans, white beans, red beans, chickpeas, lentils, grated carrot, grated courgettes, radishes, red, yellow and orange peppers, sweet corn, baby corn, sugar snap peas, mangetouts mild chillies, peas, sliced avocado, baby asparagus, cold cooked brown rice, couscous, bulgur wheat or quinoa, sliced mushrooms artichoke hearts, olives, roasted vegetables.

Consider – a little cold cooked skinless chicken or turkey, cold sliced skinless duck or game, a few crispy bacon bits, lean cooked meats, Swiss cheeses (cubed, sliced or grated), feta cheese goats cheese, cottage cheese, cooked peeled prawns, flaked fish anchovies, sardines, fresh or tinned tuna, crab or salmon, sliced or chopped boiled egg or whole quails eggs.

To Finish – slug of extra virgin olive oil or nut/seed oil, lemon or lime juice, balsamic, red or white wine vinegar, sea salt flakes ground black pepper, soy sauce, fresh nuts (whole, toasted chopped or flaked), seeds, natural yoghurt or cottage cheese wholegrain mustard, crushed garlic or ginger, drizzle of honey spoonful of fruity/spicy chutney or creamed horseradish, spoonful of peanut butter, tahini, hummus or tzatziki, shake of chilli or curry powder, Worcestershire sauce, Tabasco, tomato puree, sprinkling of chopped herbs.

NB: If you are taking a salad to work, school or you are out and about, keep the dressing separate and add just before devouring.

If you are going for shop bought salads:-

Keep all the above guidelines in mind, ensure that leafy greens and fresh vegetables form at least 50% of the mix and if not, bulk the salad out with an extra green/vegetable salad and whenever possible bin the little packet of dressing that is often included and loaded with sugar and add your own oil/lemon juice/vinegar or do without.

Quick Fix Salads with your Evening Meal
(no starchy carbohydrates included)

If you have time to make your own:-

Base – all kinds of lettuce, spinach leaves, watercress, rocket, fresh parsley and mixed herbs, sliced fennel, spring onions, sliced red onions, Chinese leaves, bok choy, mustard cress, baby gem lettuce, chicory leaves, celery leaves, chives, shredded cabbage, celery, finely sliced leeks.

Next – tomatoes (fresh and sun-dried), cucumber, bean sprouts, green beans, grated carrot, grated courgettes, radishes, red, yellow and orange peppers, sugar snap peas, mangetouts, mild chillies, peas, sliced avocado, baby asparagus, sliced mushrooms, artichoke hearts, olives, roasted vegetables.

Consider – a little cold cooked skinless chicken or turkey, cold sliced skinless duck or game, a few crispy bacon bits, lean cooked meats, Swiss cheeses (cubed, sliced or grated), feta cheese, goats cheese, cottage cheese, cooked peeled prawns, flaked fish, anchovies, sardines, fresh or tinned tuna, crab or salmon, sliced or chopped boiled egg or whole quails eggs.

To Finish – slug of extra virgin olive oil or nut/seed oil, lemon or lime juice, balsamic, red or white wine vinegar, sea salt flakes, ground black pepper, soy sauce, fresh nuts (whole, toasted, chopped or flaked), seeds, natural yoghurt or cottage cheese, wholegrain mustard, crushed garlic or ginger, drizzle of honey, spoonful of creamed horseradish, spoonful of peanut butter, tahini, hummus or tzatziki, shake of chilli or curry powder, Worcestershire sauce,

Tabasco, tomato puree, sprinkling of chopped herbs.

If you are going for shop bought salads:-

Keep all the above guidelines in mind, ensure that leafy greens and fresh vegetables form at least 50% of the mix and if not, bulk it out with an extra bag of green leafies and as recommended for your lunchtime salad, bin the ready-made dressing and make your own using some of the following:-

- extra virgin olive oil
- flax seed oil
- nut and seed oils
- avocado oil
- lemon or lime juice
- balsamic, red or white wine vinegar
- a dollop of hummus
- a dollop of cottage cheese or natural yoghurt
- a spoonful of wholegrain mustard or creamed horseradish
- a spoonful of nut butter
- crushed garlic and/or grated fresh ginger
  ...and top with a few toasted nuts or seeds

Quick Fix Snacks

- Couple of oatcakes with a slice of ham and a slice of goats' cheese cheddar.
- One sesame seed Ryvita with almond butter and sliced tomato.
- One slice of rye toast with mackerel pate and sliced cucumber.
- A small pot of natural yoghurt (*0% Total Greek*) with a handful of berries and toasted flaked almonds.
- A small pot of natural cottage cheese with fresh pineapple, mango and papaya slices.
- Couple of melon boats wrapped in Parma ham slices.
- *V8* or carrot juice and a couple of oatcakes with nut butter.
- A bowl of no-sugar muesli mix with nuts and seeds (no dried fruit) with soya/rice milk.
- Pickled herrings with rye toast soldiers.

- Soya milk latte.
- A tray of raw baby vegetables with hummus, tzatziki, natural yoghurt, cottage cheese, salsa or guacamole.
- Small pack of unsalted nuts or nuts and seeds.
- A couple of Ryvita with chopped, boiled egg (mix in a little natural yoghurt and chopped fresh herbs).
- A couple of mini oatcakes with tinned salmon and cucumber.
- A nut or nut/seed bar (no dried fruit). The *Food Doctor* and *Gillian McKeith's* are good choices.
- A couple of fresh celery sticks filled with nut butter.
- A cold boiled egg and a couple of slices of cooked ham.
- A cold, cooked chicken leg/breast (skin removed), a couple of tomatoes and a small handful of fresh nuts.
- A small pack of mixed olives with feta cheese cubes or a small bowl of olives stuffed with anchovies or almonds.
- 3 bean salad from the 'deli' section of most supermarkets.
- Half an avocado stuffed with salsa and topped with pine nuts.
- A small tray of mixed fish and vegetable sushi.
- A bowl of mixed fresh berries with shelled pistachios thrown over.
- A small pot of natural cottage cheese with sliced fresh pear and lots of black pepper.
- A slice of Pumpernickel bread toasted, spread with tzatziki and topped with thinly sliced smoked salmon and some cucumber or avocado slices.

Quick Fix Meals

Fish Fillets Thai-Style
30 mins/serves 2

Ingredients

2 fish fillets, each weighing about 140g
a small knob of fresh root ginger, peeled and chopped
1 small garlic clove, chopped
1 small red chilli, de-seeded and finely chopped
grated zest and juice of 1 lime
3 baby bok choy, each quartered lengthways
2 tbsp soy sauce

Method

1. Nestle the fish fillets side by side on a large square of foil and scatter the ginger, garlic, chilli and lime zest over them.
2. Drizzle the lime juice on top and then scatter the pieces of bok choy around and on top of the fish.
3. Pour the soy sauce over the bok choy and loosely seal the foil to make a package, making sure you leave space at the top for the steam to circulate as the fish cooks.
4. Steam for 15 mins. (If you haven't got a steamer, put the parcel on a heat-proof plate over a pan of gently simmering water, cover with a lid and steam).

Tomato, Squash and Spinach Curry
30 mins/serves 2

Ingredients

1 tbsp olive oil
1 small onion, finely sliced
1 tbsp madras curry paste
½ small butternut squash, peeled and cut into chunks
3 tomatoes, quartered
50g spinach leaves, roughly chopped

Method

1. Sauté the onion in the oil until softened.
2. Add the curry paste and cook for a further 3 mins.
3. Add the squash, tomatoes and 100ml water, stir well.
4. Cover and simmer for around 15 mins until the squash is just cooked and the tomatoes have broken down.
5. Stir through the spinach and leave for a couple of minutes to wilt.
6. Season to taste.

Beef/Lamb Stew

30 mins/serves 2

Ingredients

1 small onion, finely sliced
1 small garlic clove, finely sliced
1 tbsp olive oil
150g beef/lamb stirfry strips
½ yellow pepper, de-seeded and thinly sliced
200g chopped tomatoes
Small sprig rosemary, chopped
Heaped tbsp pitted black olives

Method

1. In a medium-sized pan, sauté onion and garlic in olive oil until softened.
2. Add beef/lamb, pepper, tomatoes and rosemary, bring to the boil then turn down the heat.
3. Simmer for 15 mins until the meat is cooked through, adding some boiling water if necessary.
4. Stir through the olives and serve.

Vegetarian alternative:
Leave out the meat and cook ½ chopped aubergine and ½ chopped courgette along with the pepper. Top with feta cheese cubes.

Turkey Burgers
25 mins/serves 2

Ingredients

250g turkey mince
Pinch dried thyme or 1 tsp fresh, chopped
½ lemon
Sea salt and freshly ground black pepper

For the relish:
100g cooked peeled beetroot (not in vinegar), finely diced
½ small red onion, very finely chopped
1 tbsp finely chopped parsley
1 tsp olive oil
1 tsp wholegrain mustard
Little gem lettuce to serve

Method

1. Put turkey into a bowl with the thyme.
2. Finely grate in the zest from the lemon and add a little seasoning.
3. Use your hands to mix the ingredients well, then shape into 2 patties.
4. Chill until ready to cook (can be frozen for up to 1 month).
5. Mix the beetroot with the juice from the lemon, onion, parsley, oil and mustard.
6. Grill or barbecue the burgers for about 6 mins each side and serve with the beetroot relish and lettuce.

Spicy Prawns
20 mins/serves 2

Ingredients

1 small onion, finely chopped
1 tsp sesame oil
1 tsp turmeric
2 garlic cloves, crushed

2cm piece fresh ginger, grated
2 tsp chilli flakes
400g tin chopped tomatoes
200g raw peeled prawns
1 tbsp low fat yoghurt

Method

1. Sauté the onion in the oil until soft.
2. Add the turmeric, garlic, ginger and chilli flakes and keep cooking for a few minutes until you end up with a rough, fragrant paste.
3. Add the tomatoes and simmer for 10 mins, adding a splash of water if required.
4. Stir in the prawns and cook until pink.
5. Serve with a dollop of yoghurt.

Beef Stroganoff

30 mins/serves 2

Ingredients

1 tbsp olive oil
1 red onion, chopped
2 garlic cloves, chopped
1 tsp paprika
1 green pepper, de-seeded and sliced
200g mushrooms, sliced
2 tbsp red wine vinegar
1 tsp *Marigold Vegetable Bouillon* powder in 150ml hot water
200g lean rump/minute steak, sliced and all fat removed
150ml *0% Total Greek* yoghurt

Method

1. Heat the oil in a pan and sauté the onion for a few mins, until soft.
2. Add the garlic and paprika and cook for 1-2 mins.
3. Add the pepper and mushrooms and sauté for 5-8 mins until softened.

4. Add the vinegar, boil to reduce until almost evaporated, then pour over the stock and bubble for a few mins until thickened slightly.
5. Add the beef and cook for 2-5 mins depending on how rare you like it. Remove from heat and leave to rest for 1-2 mins before stirring in the yoghurt gradually, to prevent splitting.
6. Season to taste.

Frittata
40 mins/serves 2

Ingredients

100g spinach, coarse stalks removed
3 eggs, lightly beaten
Pinch freshly grated nutmeg, plus a little extra
1 tsp olive oil
½ clove garlic, very finely chopped
1 handful frozen peas, defrosted
75g ricotta cheese, broken into chunks
15g finely grated parmesan
Watercress leaves, to serve

Method

1. Put the spinach in a pan with the water left clinging to the leaves after washing.
2. Cover and cook on a low heat for about 2 mins, until the spinach has completely wilted.
3. Leave to cool then squeeze out all the water, using your hands. Chop the spinach coarsely.
4. Season the beaten eggs with a little salt and freshly ground black pepper and the pinch of nutmeg.
5. Warm ½ tsp oil in a moderately hot frying pan, add the eggs and leave to cook on a low heat.
6. Meanwhile, warm the remaining ½ tsp of oil in another pan, add the spinach, garlic and peas and cook quickly until the garlic and peas are cooked and any remaining moisture has evaporated.

7. Season to taste with salt and pepper if required.
8. Dot the spinach mixture over the cooking eggs and add the ricotta. Grate some more nutmeg on top.
9. Cook for another couple of minutes then scatter the parmesan over the top.
10. Slide the frittata onto a large plate, then return it to the pan so that the uncooked side is now at the bottom. Cook for a further 5 mins or until the frittata is set. Slide onto a plate and serve with watercress leaves on the side.

Very Quick Chicken (serves 1)

Steam a skinless chicken breast either on a plate (cover it loosely with tinfoil/greaseproof paper) over a pot of simmering water or in a steam basket for 10-15 mins until cooked through. Spread pesto or olive paste on top and put under the grill (low heat) for a couple of mins until bubbling.

Very Quick Salmon (serves 1)

Lightly paint a salmon fillet or salmon steak with olive oil and grill under a moderate heat for 7-8 mins, turning once. Sprinkle with Worcestershire sauce or balsamic vinegar and lime or lemon juice just before serving.

Very Quick Fish (serves 1)

Grill or microwave a couple of white fish fillets until fish flakes easily (4-6 mins dependent on type/thickness of fish). Warm through a couple of tablespoons of tomato salsa while the fish is cooking. Top the fish with the salsa and sprinkle with chopped herbs, ground black pepper and lemon juice at the last minute.

Very Quick Lamb (serves 1)

Rub a lamb steak with lemon zest and a pinch of cinnamon mixed with a splash of olive oil. Grill under a moderate heat for 4 mins each side if you like it pink, longer for well done. Put on a warm plate and leave to rest for a few minutes while you heat through a little fresh orange juice with very finely diced red chilli then pour this over the lamb.

Very Quick Pork (serves 1)

Mix a tablespoon of peanut butter with a little sweet chilli sauce and season with pepper. Put 2 thinly sliced pork fillets on a baking tray, brush the tops with half the nutty mixture and grill under a moderate heat for 2 mins. Carefully turn the pork over, brush the other side with the remaining mixture, then grill for another 2 mins or until just cooked through. Serve with fresh apple slices and chopped fresh coriander and/or mint.

Very Quick Mackerel (serves 1)
Bake a couple of smoked mackerel fillets (skin side down) in a medium hot oven until deliciously hot and smokey. About 4-5 mins.

Very Quick Prawns (serves 1)
Coat half a dozen fresh prawns with chilli, garlic or lemon-infused olive oil and grill both sides until pink but not dried out, 2-6 mins depending on the size of the prawns.

Very Quick Omelette (serves 1)
Preheat the oven to 375F/190C/gas mark 5 and lightly grease a small baking dish with olive oil. Beat 2 eggs in a bowl and add stuff from the fridge (see below for suggestions). Season with sea salt and black pepper and pour into the prepared dish. Bake for 15-20 minutes or until the top is slightly golden and a knife inserted in the middle comes out clean. Let it cool for a few minutes before serving.

- diced cold ham
- diced cold cooked chicken
- diced Swiss cheese
- sweet peppers/artichokes/sun-dried tomatoes in jars
- freshly chopped parsley/basil
- whatever you have in stock!

Very Quick Tofu (serves 1)
Cut firm tofu into cubes and stir fry quickly in a little olive oil mixed with crushed garlic and grated fresh ginger. Add a squeeze of runny honey and top with toasted flaked almonds.

Very Quick Burger (serves 1)
Use freshly ground lean beef or soya mince which has been soaked as per packet instructions. Add some sea salt crystals, ground

black pepper and other spices of choice (cumin, coriander, curry powder, chilli powder etc), plus a few shakes of Worcestershire sauce or balsamic vinegar. Mould into patties and chill for 15 mins before grilling. Top with a slice of goats' cheese cheddar towards the end of cooking until melted and bubbling.

Quick Fix Vegetables

If you have time, pick vegetables that are in their most natural state, scrub them well or peel if absolutely necessary and know that you are getting lots of fat burning fibre, vitamins and minerals plus a wealth of protective antioxidants.

If your life is a constant rush, go for frozen vegetables which retain much of the above properties or ready to cook bags which don't pack the same nutritional punch but still deliver lots of goodness.

Steam or microwave them, make sure they retain their colour, still have a bit of bite to them and look enticing on the plate. Keep stabbing them with a sharp knife to ensure they don't overcook.

Roast or bake them if you have time and bring out the deep flavours. Cut them into big chunks, coat lightly with oil, season with salt, pepper and finely chopped or dried herbs and turn regularly (if some cook more quickly than others, just remove them while the others cook through and pop them back in for the last couple of minutes).

Grate or slice them finely and stir fry very quickly in a teaspoon or two of oil for a delicious base to many dishes.

Make them exciting and even more delicious by adding some of the following towards the end of cooking or just before serving:-

- a splash of vinegar
- a drizzle of honey
- a little marmalade or jam
- toasted nuts and/or seeds
- herb and spice mixes in oil
- a few drops of soy or fish sauce

- finely chopped parsley, basil, mint or coriander
- a few finely chopped sun-dried tomatoes or grilled peppers and some of their oil
- a drizzle of nut or seed oil

...experiment and please keep me posted on my blog/website

Quick Fix Treats

These won't do much damage as long as you regard them as treats and not as regulars when you are in the *fast lane* but should only be included when you are close to your fat loss goal (or if you are really struggling without sugar before then). Also, see *The Quick Fix Rescue Plan* for a few sweet treat choices that won't do too much harm.

- Muffins, waffles and pancakes – buy the whole grain packet mixes and top with low fat soft cheese and no sugar jam/jelly.
- Dried fruit poached in tea with a little runny honey.
- Fresh fruit dipped in 70% dark melted chocolate.
- Berry compotes (watch the sugar content).
- Halved peaches filled with crushed amaretti biscuits, drizzled with honey then grilled.
- Fruit crumbles (use muesli mixes, a little butter and honey for topping).
- Plates of chopped, sliced and whole fruits with slices of cheese (ricotta, feta, parmesan) drizzled with balsamic vinegar.
- Dates filled with pecans, almonds or walnuts.
- French toast topped with poached or fresh fruit.
- Home made or good quality bought carrot cake, banana cake or fruit loaf (lose the icing).

Quick Fix Drinks

- Water, of course but it can get a bit dull so opt for the sparkling version from time to time and add lots of ice, fresh strawberries, fresh lime, cucumber, fresh mint and a splash of fresh fruit cordial.
- Black, green, red bush or fruit/herb tea without milk or sugar

Try them chilled on crushed ice, topped up with water and add a spoonful of honey and some fresh lemon/lime juice.

- Good quality coffee from ground beans with no milk or sugar. Do it the European way and have a large glass of water alongside. Have a soya latte/cappuccino with no sugar occasionally if you are feeling seriously deprived.
- A glass or two of rich red or dry white wine.
- A Bloody Mary or a Bloody Caesar (with clam juice) or a Virgin Mary - very tall glass, lots of ice, lots of seasoning and a large stick of celery.

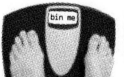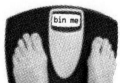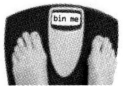

Part 6. The Quick Fix Rescue Plan

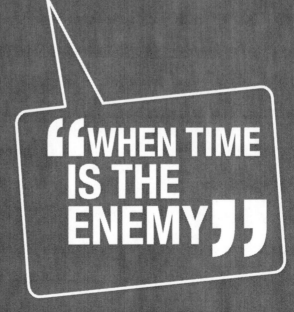

"WHEN TIME IS THE ENEMY"

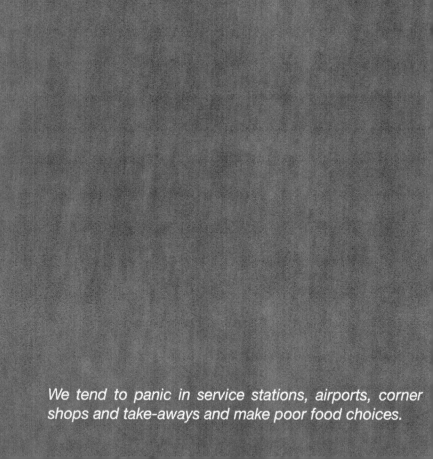

We tend to panic in service stations, airports, corner shops and take-aways and make poor food choices.

The Quick Fix Rescue Plan

Top food choices when time is the enemy and continued fat loss is threatened.

Things can go horribly wrong for dieters when you haven't eaten for a few hours, hunger strikes and you haven't planned ahead. Rather too many studies indicate that we tend to panic in mini supermarkets, service stations, airports, railway stations, corner shops or take-aways and we either make poor choices or eat nothing. Neither route helps fat loss, so rescue tactics are vital.

Regard this section of the book as an ally, photocopy it from the book or download it from my website and keep it near you at all times; it will seriously limit potential damage. Some of the suggestions are not 100% in tune with the *2 Weeks in the Fast Lane Plan* but they will help you stay on track.

Sandwiches, Wraps and Baguettes

- Go for brown bread, rolls or baguettes, the denser the better and take the top off to form an open sandwich.
- If a single sandwich is on offer, grab it (half the damage of a 2 pack).
- Pick the ones that are jam-packed with salad or vegetables.
- Opt for fresh or tinned salmon, crab, tuna, beef, lamb, chicken or beans/chickpeas so you get a decent amount of protein to fill you up quickly.
- If it looks creamy there's likely too much mayonnaise, avoid them if you can.
- If you prefer a wrap, unwrap it, grab a fork, eat the contents and bin most of the wrap.
- In a *pick your own fillings* establishment, get them to box your selection and ignore the roll.

Soups

- Thick soups are best when you are ravenous because they fill the void quickly.
- Soups with beans, lentils, chickpeas, peas, broad beans, sweet potato or butternut squash involved won't do anything like the damage of those packed with the white stuff (potato, pasta or rice).
- Asian-style soups are generally fine because they include fat burning spices. Coconut milk is often involved but is a better choice than cows milk or cream because it is richer in healthy fats. Many are bulked up with noodles or rice but if you sup the soup and leave the starchy carbohydrates at the bottom of the pot you won't go far wrong.
- If you opt for a vegetable soup, grab a small pack of fresh nuts or nuts and seeds to have on the side so you get some protein to ensure hunger doesn't return all too quickly.

Snacks

- **Nuts and seeds** are packed with protein, fat burning and filling good fats and can't be beaten when hunger strikes. But, to ensure you don't hoover a huge bag in one go buy small packs, add a piece of fresh fruit and a chunk of cheese.
- **Salty snacks** deliver little other than quick but short-lived satisfaction but if there is little else on offer you can limit the damage by opting for a small bag and scoffing a few slices of pre-packed ham, chicken, beef, corned beef or tongue.
- **Cheese** can pile on the pounds if consumed regularly and in copious amounts but it can be a great hunger-buster if you make the right choices. Portioned and small packs are available everywhere. Go for hard cheeses, Swiss cheese, goats' cheese and ewes' milk cheeses to reduce the saturated fat content. Better still have a pot of cottage

cheese (go for the ones with added extras or throw in a small pack of nuts and raisins if you are not a big cottage cheese fan).

- **Tinned fish** can be a bit messy and smelly, but salmon, sardines, anchovies, mackerel, crab or pilchards squashed onto a couple of Ryvitas will fill you up quickly.
- **Oats** are great when you are hungry. It's not hard to find a tub of ready made porridge or a cereal bar rich in oats and whilst many are overly-laced with sugar they are still a better choice than a burger and chips or a BLT. If you can get your hands on a packet of oatcakes, some hummus and a few baby tomatoes so much the better.
- **Fruit** is a morning (and on its own) requirement on the *fast lane* plan but if there is little else available, no matter what time of day, grab it. Fresh, dried, with nuts, in a smoothie or yoghurt or in a salad mix is always going to be a better choice than a ham and cheese panini.
- **Sweet treats** do little to nourish the body, they merely feed our desires. So, how do we feed the desire without straying too far from the fat loss path? **Small is beautiful** - a kids' sized bar of chocolate will deliver the sugar hit with less than half the sugar of a standard bar. And, stay away from low fat treats, they often have more sugar than the original versions. Look out for the following when it's got to be sugar:-

  - mini bar of dark chocolate (70% cocoa solids)
  - slice of carrot cake (bin the icing)
  - slice of banana loaf
  - slice of fruit cake (bin the icing)
  - small frozen yoghurt
  - fruit, nut and seed bars
  - a fruit scone
  - a bran muffin
  - a kids' pack of chocolate buttons
  - a few dates filled with pecans or almonds
  - a small fruit yoghurt

- a pack of 2 shortbread fingers
- a small packet of wine gums

Main Dishes

- **Italian:** Selection of cold meats/cheeses, chicken or meatballs in tomato/pepper sauce, mixed fresh salads. Body swerve pasta and potatoes and if it has to be pizza go for the thinnest base, go easy on the cheese and make sure it is stacked to the gunnels with vegetables and fish or chicken.
- **Indian:** Poppadoms with spicy onions, dhal, kebabs with yoghurt/cucumber sauce, tandoori chicken, lamb or beef with a little sweet/sour sauce on the side. Say no to the rice and naan bread.
- **Chinese:** Egg drop soup, hot and sour soup, prawns with ginger and spring onion, satay chicken, pork or beef, bean casseroles, stir fried vegetables. Avoid anything with noodles or rice or leave them on the side.
- **French:** Onion Soup (bin the cheesy crouton), soup provençal (lots of vegetables in there), tuna niçoise salad, coq au vin, mussels marinière, beef bourguignon. Ask for extra vegetables/salad and don't have mash, potatoes dauphinoise or frites.
- **Burger Places:** Go for a plain burger, ketchup and mustard on the side won't hurt, no need for the bun or the fries and get them to sling as much salad into the box as they can.
- **The Kebab Shop:** not a great choice for fat loss but if it's your only option refuse the pitta, ask them to put lots of salad in a box with grilled chicken and top it with the yoghurt dressing.
- **Pie and Pasty Shops:** don't go there - find an alternative!

Other Dangerous Situations

- **In a bar:** Ask for a bowl of olives and/or fresh nuts if they are available or go next door to the corner shop if there is one and grab a leg of chicken or a packet of processed meat and wolf some down quickly. Salty snacks on the bar are way too moreish when you are having a drink and you haven't eaten for a while. Even a bit of *plastic* cheese will stem the need for these diet disrupters.
- **Room service:** When you arrive at a hotel and you are tired and hungry it's hard to stick with the programme if you haven't planned ahead and room service is your only option. Go for a steak, grilled chicken or fish with lots of vegetables or salad if you are there early enough but if it's late the menu is often limited to a Caesar Salad, bit too much mayo but not a bad choice, a burger and chips (ask for no bun, no fries and lots of salad), some sort of chicken and rice dish (ask for more chicken, sauce etc and lose the rice), a club sandwich (see if they might be willing to give you all the filling on top of just one slice of toast) or if you are lucky, a plain or filled omelette. No matter how poor the selection they always have salad to hand so ask nicely and you can get lucky! There are also things the staff can be coerced into adding to the tray like olives and nuts which can help to satisfy your appetite. Always worth a try!
- **On a plane:** If you haven't planned ahead and you are on a long-haul flight it can be tricky. Your best bet is to drink loads of water, get fresh and dried fruit and nut snacks whenever the trolley passes by and when the meals arrive, eat the protein and stay away from the bread, potatoes, crackers, biscuits and cakes. If it's a short flight have a tomato juice and a packet of fresh nuts and if you are still hungry at the other end, grab a healthy snack at the airport so you are not hungry and tempted to gorge when you get to your final destination.

- **On the road:** If you spend a lot of your day on motorways you are sorted as many of them now have mini supermarkets where you can pick up some great and healthy snacks to keep you going. But, if you are restricted to service stations and roadside eateries it gets a whole lot more difficult when you are on a fat loss plan and you don't have any snacks or lunch with you. However, you can usually get a breakfast anywhere at any time of the day. Ask for eggs (scrambled, boiled or poached but not fried), a couple of rashers of bacon (cut the fat off), grilled tomatoes and mushrooms and baked beans. Don't be coerced into the sausages, fried bread, black pudding and toast on the side. A healthier version of the Great British Breakfast will keep you nourished for hours and you need only top up with some fresh fruit and a packet of nuts later in the day and not too much damage will have been done.

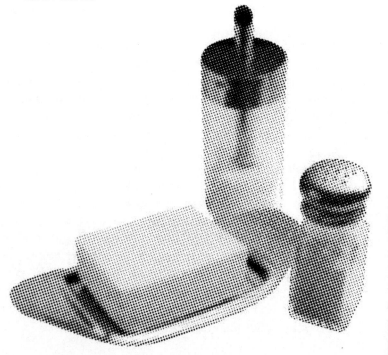

Glossary of Terms

A

Absorption: the process by which nutrients are taken from the intestines into the bloodstream then into body cells.

Acidic: having a pH of less than 7.

Adrenaline: a hormone that is produced by the adrenal gland when stress or danger is sensed by the body. It increases blood pressure, heart rate and blood flow to muscles.

Aerobic: requiring oxygen.

Amino Acids: the basic building blocks from which proteins are assembled. There are eight essential amino acids which must be derived from the protein foods we eat to enable the body to rebuild and repair.

Anaerobic: the absence of oxygen or the absence of a need for oxygen.

Antioxidants: dietary substances capable of neutralising free radicals which in excess, could otherwise cause damage to body tissue and lead to cell dysfunction.

B

Body Mass Index (BMI): a measure of body fat.

Basal Metabolic Rate (BMR): The metabolic rate as measured under basal conditions, 12 hours after eating, after a restful sleep, no exercise or activity preceding test, elimination of emotional excitement and occurring in a comfortable temperature.

C

Calorie: a unit of measurement of energy. One calorie is defined as the amount of energy required to raise one cubic centimetre of water by one degree centigrade.

Cardiovascular: referring to the heart and blood vessels.

Cell Membrane: the barrier that separates the contents of a body cell from its outside environment and controls what moves in and out of the cell.

D

Detoxification: the process of getting rid of toxic matter from the body.

Diabetes Mellitus: a chronic metabolic disease characterised by abnormally high blood glucose (sugar) levels, resulting from the inability of the body to produce or respond to insulin.

Diuretic: an agent that increases the formation of urine by the kidneys, resulting in water loss.

DNA: the genetic coding found in the nucleus (the brain) of every body cell which determines specific characteristics and functions within the body.

E

Electron: a stable atomic particle with a negative charge.

Enzymes: made up of a complex of amino acids, enzymes are part of every chemical reaction in living things. These include all digestion, growth and building of cells, and breakdown of substances such as vitamins and nutrients and all reactions involving the transformation of energy.

Essential Fatty Acids: linoleic acid (Omega 6s) and linolenic acid (Omega 3s) are 'essential' because the body cannot make them or work without them. They are important for brain development, controlling inflammation, blood clotting, heart health etc and must be derived from our diet.

F

Fermentation: an anaerobic process that involves the breakdown of dietary components to yield energy.

Free Radicals: highly reactive molecules possessing unpaired electrons that are produced during the metabolism of food and energy. They are believed to contribute to the molecular damage and death of vital body cells and may be a factor in ageing and disease. Antioxidants help neutralise them.

G

Gene: a region of DNA that controls a specific hereditary characteristic, usually corresponding to a single protein.

Glucagon: a hormone responsible for helping maintain balanced blood sugar levels. When blood sugar levels get too low, glucagon activates glucose production in the liver, as well as regulating the release of glycogen from muscle cells.

Glucose: a 6-carbon sugar which plays a major role in the generation of energy for living organisms.

Glycogen: a large chain of glucose molecules used to store energy in cells, especially muscle and liver cells.

H

Hormone: a chemical, released by a gland or a tissue, which affects or regulates the activity of specific cells or organs. Complex bodily functions, such as growth and sexual development are regulated by hormones.

I

Immune System: the body's defence against infectious organisms and other invaders. Through a series of steps called the immune response, the immune system attacks organisms and substances that invade body systems and cause disease.

Insulin: a hormone secreted by the beta-cells of the pancreas required for normal glucose metabolism.

M

Macronutrient: nutrients required in relatively large amounts; macronutrients include carbohydrates, protein and fats.

Malabsorption: poor absorption of nutrients from food.

Metabolism: the sum of the processes (reactions) by which a substance is taken in and incorporated into the body or detoxified and excreted from the body.

Micronutrient: a nutrient required by the body in small

amounts, such as vitamins and minerals.

Minerals: nutritionally important elements which are composed of only one kind of atom. They are inorganic (do not contain carbon as do vitamins and other organic compounds).

N

Neurotransmitter: a chemical that is released from a nerve cell and results in the transmission of an impulse to another nerve cell or organ. Dopamine and serotonin are neurotransmitters.

Nutrient: any substance that can be metabolised by a living creature to provide energy and build tissue.

O

Omega 3's: see 'Essential Fatty Acids'.

Omega 6's: see 'Essential Fatty Acids'.

Optimum Health: in addition to freedom from disease, the ability of an individual to function physically and mentally at his/her best.

Oxidation: a chemical reaction that removes electrons from an atom or molecule.

Oxidative Damage: damage to cells caused by free radicals.

P

Pancreas: a small organ located behind the stomach and connected to the small intestine. The pancreas synthesises enzymes that help digest food in the small intestine and hormones, including insulin, that regulate blood glucose levels.

Phytonutrients: compounds derived from plants in our diet.

Protein: a complex organic molecule composed of amino acids in a specific order. The order is determined by the sequence of nucleic acids in a gene coding for the protein. Proteins are required for the structure, function and regulation of body cells, tissues and organs and each protein has unique functions.

S
Satiety: refers to the feeling of satisfaction or 'fullness' produced by the consumption of food.

Saturated Fats: fatty acids with no double bonds between carbon atoms.

Small Intestine: the part of the digestive tract that extends from the stomach to the large intestine. The small intestine includes the duodenum (closest to the stomach), the jejunum and the ileum (closest to the large intestine).

Supplement: a nutrient or phytochemical supplied in addition to that which is obtained in the diet.

T
Thermogenic: production of heat.

Thyroid: a butterfly-shaped gland in the neck that secretes thyroid hormones. Thyroid hormones regulate a number of physiological processes, including growth, development, metabolism and reproductive function.

V
Vitamin: an organic (carbon-containing) compound necessary for normal physiological function that cannot be synthesised in adequate amounts and must therefore be obtained in the diet.

Index

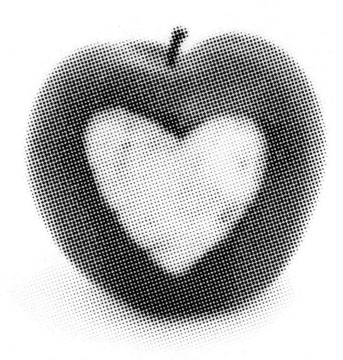

Fiona
Kirk
eat, live, love

For more information visit
www.fionakirk.com